QUALITY LIFE FOR WOMEN OVER 50

The ER Quality Life System

Quality Life for Women Over 50 - The ER Quality Life System

Research by Elizabeth Roddick
Cover Design by Kinga Stabryla
Typesetting and proofreading by Kinga Stabryla
Yoga Images by Julie Hanson

Email: hello@erqualitylifesystem.com
Facebook: CallThePharmacistUK
http://erqualitylifesystem.com

DISCLAIMER
Any information in this book is not a subsitute for medical advice. Before attempting any of the exercises you may want to consider seeking advice from a healthcare professional.

Although the author has made every effort to ensure that the information in this book was correct at the time of printing, the author does not assume and hereby disclaim any liability to any party for any loss, damage or disruption caused by errors or omissions, whether such errors or omissions result from negligence, accident, or any other cause.

This book is dedicated to older women who deserve a real quality of life as they age.

Acknowledgements

With thanks to

Nancy Van Allan

Jennifer Strong

Karen Curran

June Alexander

Jane Cameron, and

Alison McKinnon

for their helpful reviews.

CONTENTS

Introduction

Introduction

When a woman reaches 50, the modern world is all about anti-ageing. 'What about my wrinkles, my eyesight is failing and suddenly I have aches and pains where I used to be supple?' The psychological part of getting older is sometimes the hardest part to address.

Life at this time should be about a sense of freedom and good changes.

What if there was a system that gave you new ideas and allowed you to flourish into the woman you want to be? One that made you relaxed and happy in your body, but also really excited about what lies ahead? I believe you can be that woman, and I am asking you to follow the system laid out in the chapters - for you. Then, I would like you to pick out the parts that really resonate with you and see what changes can make a real difference for the better.

Why do you need a system? A system is a set of ideas, a route you can follow. Have you ever had something to learn where you did not have any information or a path to follow? In fact, it did not even make sense. How did you get on?

The ER Quality Life System contains a diverse amount of knowledge. There are 19 chapters full of information. Underpinning all this information is how you can utilise your mind to achieve the quality of life you want. I say 'you' because it is your decision. What the system means to do, by giving you ideas and facts, is open up possibilities – perhaps making you think differently about yourself.

The different chapters are designed to be relevant to someone, and I know you will find something that will help you move on. I'm excited for you!

Have a great journey!

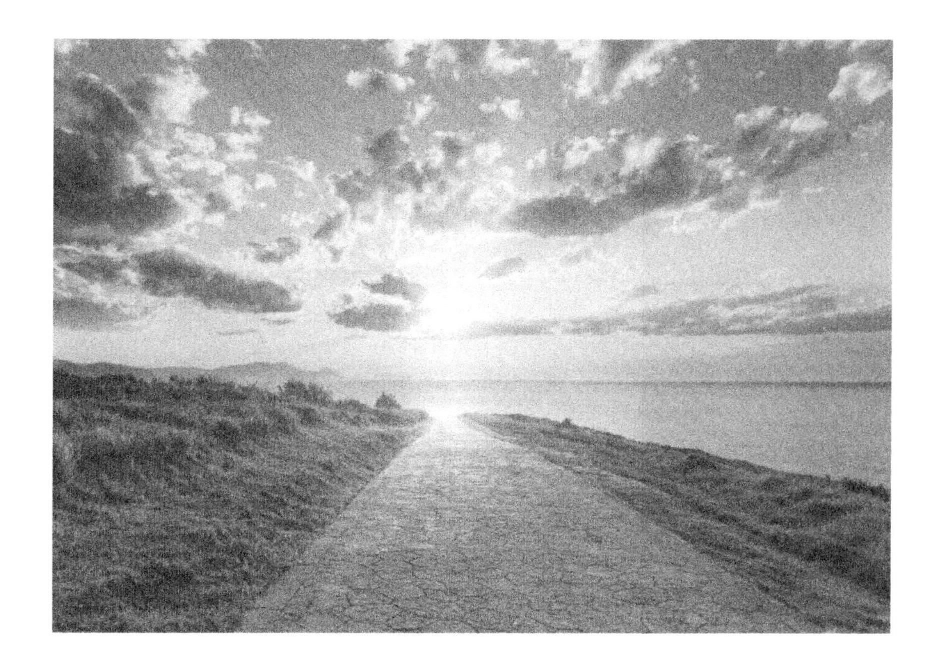

Chapter 1

E is for Easy

For something to be 'easy', you need to know how to do something and be able to follow it effortlessly. Have you heard of the expression unconscious competence? It is from a learning model developed by Martin Bradwell who published the model in the Gospel Guardian in 1969.

The example I'm going to use is that of driving a car. Think about when you drove or walked, if you don't drive, along a route to get somewhere and you didn't recollect anything about the journey? If you are in a city, you would have stopped at each set of lights or crossroads, manoeuvred around various obstacles and worryingly, may not have been aware of it. This is known as 'unconsciously competent' in the model.

The first stage is 'unconscious incompetence', in other words, you don't actually know that you don't know what to do. The next stage is 'conscious incompetence' - yes, you do now realise that you don't know how to perform something. The third stage is 'conscious competence' - you know you are competent. The last stage is the example I gave driving a car on a familiar journey and not remembering what happened at the end of the journey. It means that somehow your brain allowed you to function competently with a familiar action without having to engage your conscious mind.

I'm looking for you to be 'unconsciously competent' regarding the ER Quality Life system because it is easy to follow. I emphasise mindset in some of the chapters since it can make such a difference to the outcome.

In the Cambridge dictionary, the definition of mindset is 'a person's way of thinking and their opinions.' The best way to describe mindset is to give you an example:

Jinnie was of the firm belief that when you reach a certain age you have to behave differently than before. She had just been at her doctor's where she was asked 'what do you expect at your age?'

'So, it was right' said Jinnie 'things will just start going downhill from now on! What has my life been about?' She was starting to feel a bit depressed.

'Jinnie I want to start by asking you what you love to do?', I asked. Jinnie was a bit taken aback by that question. She thought for a minute and said 'Well, I love to delve back in history and find out why things have happened in particular countries.' 'So, how often do you do that?', I responded. 'Practically never', said Jinnie. 'You probably know my next question. Why not?', I asked.

This is where I find women come out with all sorts of excuses from children to elderly parents to partners and then, of course, work.

As an NLP practitioner (Neurolinguistic practitioner), my job is to ask questions and find out the real reasons for beliefs like 'yes, things will just go downhill from now on.' The skill is to take those beliefs, examine them and regurgitate them in a different way. My goal is for the woman to be thinking differently when she leaves. It's not enough to think that way just after a session. The thoughts need to be reinforced so that it is the new way of thinking that is permanent.

It was interesting in Jinnie's case that it had been her mother who had repeatedly stated negative beliefs about ageing. We did have a discussion about what was going on in her mother's life before she passed away. 'She had been very old fashioned. She stayed at home when my sister and I were young and seemed to be angry about her place in life. My father was the breadwinner, and he expected my mother to keep the home clean and prepare meals. She never really had time to do the things that she wanted and as she got older it was as if it was inevitable that it was going to be downhill.'

'Do you think that coloured your view of ageing?', I asked. 'Yes, it did' admitted Jinnie.

Now was the time to introduce one of the NLP techniques.

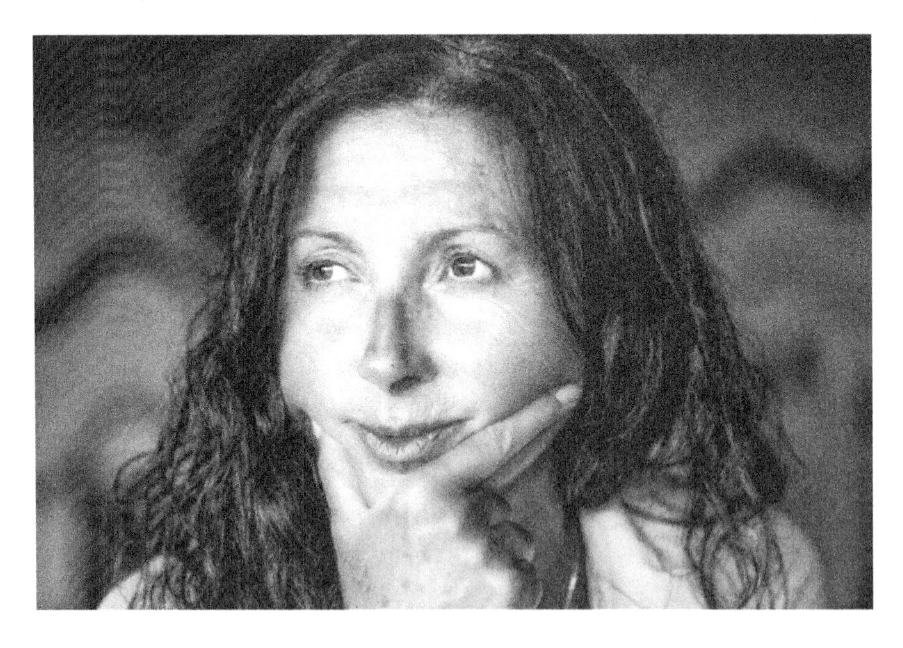

'Jinnie, I want you to imagine you are at the cinema. Right in front of you is the screen, and I want you to see a small black and white picture of your mother telling you how her own life is not worth living. And then get rid of the image, to make it a white one, and then I want you to make it much bigger. In fact, it now completely fills the space in front of you. Now I want you to add colour – beautiful colour that lifts your spirits. You see your mother smiling broadly looking younger than her years and yes, her voice has become younger, more vibrant and she is cajoling you to make the very best of your life. I want you to really hear her voice, see her bright eyes and feel that feeling of hope and positivity inside.'

This exercise had to be repeated several times but Jinnie did start to look at ageing in a different light.

TIPS FOR MAKING THINGS EASY

1. Make time for things you like to do.
2. Change your beliefs using imagination.

chapter 2

R is for Relationships

I believe relationships sometimes have to change.

Something you can reflect on - where are you now? Sometimes women live another person's life instead of their own.

Steph felt she had always lived in the shadow of her husband. He had been a C.E.O of a successful haulage firm and because it meant he was away a lot 'doing deals' on the continent, where most of the work was based, she found herself bringing up the children basically on her own. Her own dreams and, in fact, personal development had taken a back seat. All the business functions she had to attend (as she felt as an appendage) simply were beginning to rile her. Feeling unfulfilled, she confronted her husband David one night.

'David, have you ever felt, in one of your deals, that you seemed to be pushed aside and frustrated?' 'Of course,' said David 'that does happen from time to time'.

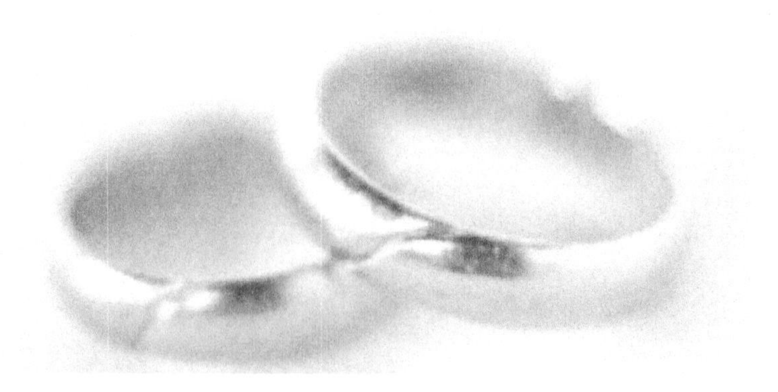

'Well can you see how I feel?' said Steph. 'It's as if I am living your life not even by your side but almost as an afterthought.'

'Wow' said David 'I had no idea that you felt that way.' There was silence for a while. Then David, rather tentatively, said 'what has to change?' He was desperately hoping that he could salvage their marriage that he now realised was in a precarious position.

Steph looked at the worried expression on her husband's face.

'It's alright, I'm not going to leave you.' said Steph.

David's body relaxed and for the first time, probably in a long time, they discussed Steph's feelings and how they could move on from where they were.

'I've written a couple of short stories. The local magazine editor has said he would like to publish them, but I need time to write. That requires changes in the way we live our lives.'

Yes, this was a very understanding husband and things did change.

Is this something you can relate to?

Loneliness, as you grow older, can be a problem that ultimately can affect health. Research has shown that on top of affecting mental health, it also affects physical health. It's interesting that psychologically, even being amongst a crowd of people can lead someone to a feeling of loneliness. Clearly, we have been through a difficult time, and you may have had that real experience.

Can you think about the relationships you have picked up over the years? Some will be lifelong friendships, others transitory, linking where you did not even realise that the link has been made. Over the years, you would have probably helped many people, even unwillingly, and many years later someone may have came back into your life to repay that kindness.

The opposite is also true. If you have caused upset to someone, they then may not ever forgive you. While I am on the subject of forgiveness, it is so important for you to do that - not necessarily in person - but, through say an unposted letter. The activity of writing such a letter where you apologise to the person or indeed forgive them is such a powerful thing to do.

Have you ever thought about your funeral? Maybe not a subject you would normally read about in a quality life self-help book but now you have the chance to steer your life the way you want it.

Sit back in your seat, close your eyes and imagine your funeral. Are there many people there? Let us look closely at the faces - are there those who are upset or those who are joking with each other before the coffin arrives?

The minister or celebrant starts to speak 'we are here to celebrate the life of..........'

This is where you have the chance to put in the words you want to hear. It may also be a time when you realise you haven't fulfilled your potential. The great thing is you now have the chance to do that.

THINK ABOUT YOUR RELATIONSHIPS

1) Do they have to change?
2) Do you have to change?
3) Do you need to find new relationships?

Chapter 3

Q is for Quality

As this system is about attaining quality in your life, I thought I would tell you about some research on the subject.

Andrade et al[1] looked at the association between frailty and family functionality on health - related quality of life. They wanted to find the physical component as well as the mental component parts in relation to family support. Interestingly, positive social interactions regarding family showed an increased quality of life.

Social support helps older people become more resilient. I remember Jean - she was a domineering woman who charged around not noticing the fact that those around her were reeling at the force of her character. One day Jean became ill. This was something she had really not encountered in her life. Illness was for weak people, not for her. Suddenly she had to rely on those people around her for normal tasks – she even had to rely on a carer to help her shower and get to the bathroom.

Reflection is a great leveler when focused on reality. Reflecting on her new life Jean became depressed and there was only one member of her family, her niece, who had stuck resolutely by her. As a result, she was able to see just what had happened in the past and perhaps what she could do now to help herself. Resilience is something that can be learned. It's not an easy trait but in Jean's case pointing out where she had been in her life and where she was now, awakened something inside. Yes, she decided that taking each day to strengthen her body allowed her to work on her mind, moving her to a new dimension where the depression lifted and she started to form new links with those around her. Resolving problems has been shown to improve the quality of life of older women.

Can you relate to Jean in any way?

I decided to do my own research and asked 30 of my female patients over 50 years of age what were the most important factors in giving them a quality of life? The research was carried out pre- pandemic, so if the same question was put to women now it probably wouldn't evoke the same answers.
I categorised the women's answers according to which decade of age they belonged to e.g., 50-60, 61-70, 71-80 and 80+.

The results were as follows:

	age 50-60	61 - 70	80+
Health	16	15	
Family	10	15	
Good eyesight		2	
Overwhelmed (no answer)			1
Time	1		
Social mixing		10	
Mobility		1	
Money (comfortable)		4	
Mentally alert		1	
Security		1	
Honesty		1	
Love of family		1	
Time to give to family		1	
Walking	1		
Good diet	1		

Reduced stress		1	
Quality sleep	2		
Washing machine/ shower	1		

As you can see, the most important factors were health and family. Do you agree?

Henchoz et al[2] looked at determinants of quality of life in community-dwelling older adults and it was found that there was a reduction in any decline of the quality of life if the individuals were able to reduce their disability and deal with any depressive symptoms.

TIPS AND THOUGHTS

1. What are the important determinants in your life regarding quality?
2. What can you do to help yourself lead that life you want?

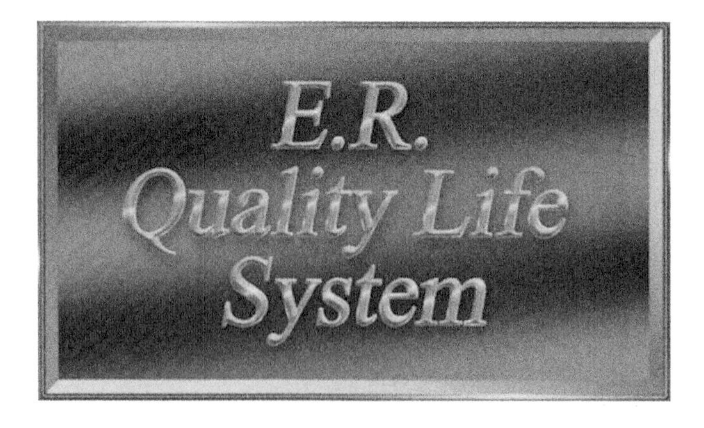

Chapter 4

U is for Understanding

Have you ever had conflicts at work or at home that just did not seem to be able to be resolved?

Sarah had a problem at work. Two of her staff had fallen out with each other over a task that neither wished to do. It was causing a very unpleasant atmosphere in the workplace and she knew it had to be resolved as quickly as possible. Let us call the two members of staff Lara and Susan - who coincidentally were two women in their 50's.

'Lara and Su' said Sarah, when she managed to get the two members of staff to stand together in front of her - not an easy task. 'At the end of work today I would like to have a meeting - just the three of us - so that we can try and resolve things. Is that o.k.?'

'Well, I don't think that's......' said Sue. Sarah interjected 'Let's just see what happens.'

6 pm arrived and the three ladies went into the staff room, Lara and Susan finding seats as far apart as possible.

'Right ladies' said Sarah 'this is what is going to happen. You are going to put your chairs so that you are facing each other. Yes, I know that is difficult just now.'

Both ladies took their chairs as instructed and very warily sat down opposite each other.

'Now' said Sarah 'the idea is that each person will have two minutes to speak about what's wrong - I'll use my phone alarm. When the alarm goes off then you must stop talking and then the other person has two minutes to speak. At no time must there be any interruptions. Is that understood?'

Both ladies nodded gravely. 'Right', said Sarah, 'I'm going to ask Lara to start because she is first in the alphabet and for no other reason. Your time starts now.'

Lara gave a full description of what had happened and how she felt so hurt by Susan.

'Right, time is up', said Sarah.

This time it was Sue's chance to give her side but instead of berating Lara, she realised what she had done - hurt her colleague. She didn't get to the two-minute mark before they were hugging each other and apologising.

No, it doesn't always work out like that, but often when you allow someone to speak without interruption then things can get resolved without the conflict. Yes, understanding is a great tool to use.

Listening skills are another very important aspect of understanding.

Have you ever been talking with someone one to one and you have noticed they keep looking over your shoulder? How does that make you feel? I have experienced that, and I felt angry at the time. You might have felt another emotion, for example disappointment, at the fact that you are possibly not seen as worthy of being given someone's full attention. Health professionals have a habit of looking at the computer instead of you.

One of the real aptitudes of listening skills is to make the person in front of you feel as if they are the most important person at that moment and they are worthy of your complete attention.

Peter Thomson, an entrepreneur, talks about listening so intently that inside your head you repeat the words you are hearing, then speak back to the person in their own words. This is a skill that you need to practice, otherwise it sounds very contrived. But once you master it, it can be one of the most powerful communication skills in your toolbox.

Derek was seventeen years old and prided himself on being popular at school and he knew he would always be accepted as 'one of the lads'. The problem was that his popularity meant he thought of himself as above any rules that were made at home for him to follow.

One of the rules was to be in the house by a certain time at night. He flouted the rules almost every night and, although his parents tried to demand that he followed them, nothing was working.

Tanya had been talking to her friend one night, Jilly, when she came across a technique that seemed to work certainly with Jilly and her daughter Sharon. (This is similar to the technique mentioned in chapter 2 Relationships). The technique involves taking an example in your son's or daughter's life and how they feel about that and relating it back to how you feel about their behaviour.

'Derek, I wanted to ask you a question', said Tanya. Immediately Derek's eyes rolled and he silently thought 'here we go again'. 'You know how you are desperate to play the lead in the school production this year?' 'Yes', said Derek wondering where this was going. 'Well, how does that make you feel when you are always chosen for the chorus rather than the leading man?'

Derek thought for a minute. 'Pretty angry and frustrated actually'. 'Well, I want you to hang onto that feeling and imagine how myself and your father feel when you don't follow the rules at night.'

Suddenly the dark clouds lifted, and Derek started to smile. 'Well, if you put it that way maybe I need to think about these rules.'

Did it make a difference? Yes - not every night, but it was certainly a vast improvement on what had been happening before.

Maybe you don't have teenage children, maybe it's grown-up children or a boss at work. By using this analogy based on feelings you can help someone understand how you feel.

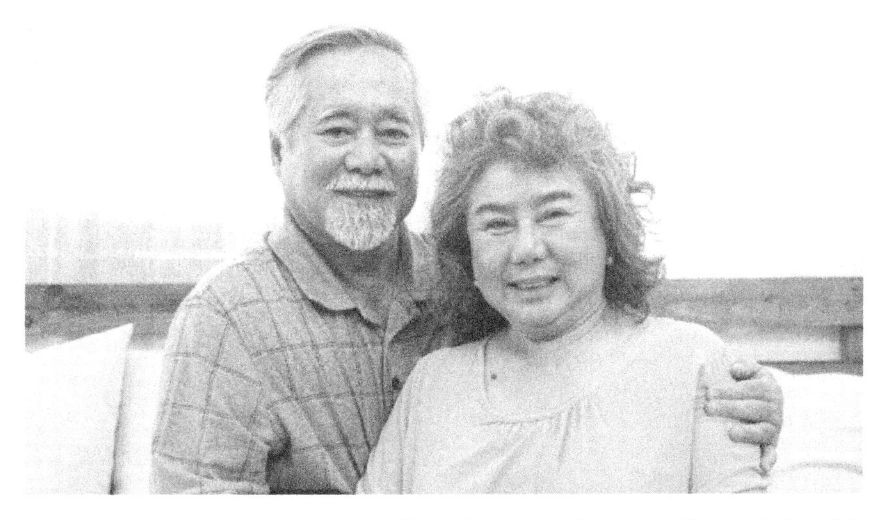

TIPS AND THOUGHTS

1. Is understanding a scenario or person in relation to yourself something you need to resolve?
2. Look at the examples - can you adapt one to your own life?

Chapter 5

A is for Age

Have you heard the expression age is just a number?

How old are you? Does it matter? I think as soon as you tell someone your age you are immediately placed in a box, yet that doesn't have to be. Researchers in America decided to take a group of 80-year-olds and immerse them in an environment reflecting when they were in their 40's. This meant that music was played from that era. Pictures on the wall reflected what was going on at the time and newspapers had the dates of those years as well. When the older people sat down to a meal, it was first of all, sitting at a table on a chair from that vintage. Also, the wallpaper was of that time and the food they were eating was the sort of food they would have prepared in their kitchens. In fact, some of them were made to make their own meals - something they hadn't done for some time.

Each of them was brought to a place where they either used to work or go to the cinema to stimulate a youthful memory. What they found was that the men and women had improved cognitive function, memory and physical markers, such as strength. Why was that?

The researcher's conclusion was that immersing an individual in an environment that depicted an era when they felt at their peak and invigorated then this somehow had a beneficial effect on the psychology of ageing.

I sometimes think when I see grandparents interacting with their grandchildren they become 'child like' and take on the persona of a much younger person.

Experiments have been done within residential homes where they introduce toddlers into the home to interact with the residents. Again, what is astonishing, is, that even those with a degree of dementia show some signs of improvement.

On the negative side, society sometimes sidelines older individuals. Avril was at the front of the queue in the bakery. Behind the counter was a youngish man serving. He raised his head, looked through Avril and asked the gentleman behind if he could help! Avril immediately intervened: 'Sorry, I was here first' where the server looked at Avril without any apology 'Yes, what is it you want?'

Another example was where an experiment was conducted using an actress. The actress was a 31-year-old attractive lady. She dressed up in old fashioned clothes with a headscarf and the makeup department had created an older looking face using ageing techniques on skin.

The shop was a greengrocer and, as the older woman gathered items into her basket, she went forward to pay but struggled to get money from her purse. The server, instead of helping, went on to serve another customer with frustration showing in her face.

The next day, the actor was herself. She had a long mane of auburn hair, up to date nails, makeup and wearing a smart pink suit. The difference in attendance was staggering. The actor once again was seen struggling with getting money from a purse but this time everything was put on hold while the server made comments like:

'Yes, sometimes it's difficult to get the money out – just take your time.'

Does society, in general, treat older women differently?

I want to tell you about Tanya. Being from an ethnic minority she had always struggled to fit in at school and that struggle more or less plagued her life. She had, however, done well at school, attained a first-class honours degree in law and has become a very successful barrister.

She didn't feel successful though and at 60 years old she realised the sort of life she had been leading had not been true to herself. Although this was apart from anything she had done before, she decided to consult a hypnotist. The hypnotist was very skilful with language allowing Tanya to go back in time to see where this feeling of insecurity or 'not being good enough' had come from. She traced it back to her father who had somehow undermined her accomplishments all of her life and never given her even an inkling of any pride he had in her.

'Why should I live my life in his shadow?' she remarked after the first session. The hypnotist then gradually built up Tanya's confidence so that at the end of the third session she was true to herself.

I think it is very important for women to be comfortable in their own skins. The problem is I know many who are not. My late mother, for example, had an anger inside that manifested in outbursts of rage resulting from never being at peace with herself.

Being at peace with yourself is an important aspect of the system and if you do not find all the answers here then I can help you find them.

Do you know the difference between your chronological age and your biological one?

Researchers have wrestled with different markers and biochemical markers are sometimes used but below are general statements:

Aerobic capacity

Aerobic means with oxygen. How quickly do you run out of breath? This can be measured by wearing breathing apparatus and running on a treadmill. The fitter you are the better your aerobic capacity will be.

Antioxidant levels

Antioxidant levels are a measure of your age since it declines markedly from your youth. Remember how quickly you healed as a child? Many older people have wounds that simply don't heal.

Auditory acuity

Do you have to turn up the television these days? The higher definition on the auditory scale starts to decline with age. When you go for a hearing check it's often found that auditory sharpness has declined.

Blood pressure

I remember listening to a lecture by an eminent researcher (it was at the Edinburgh Science Festival where I was hosting a session on vitamin D). An audience member asked a question about covering up skin to protect from cancer. He replied that she would have a far greater risk of dying of high blood pressure. He then went on to say that when the skin is exposed to the sun it produces nitrous oxide which in turn reduces blood pressure. Your blood pressure naturally rises with age. A 20-year-old woman might have a blood pressure of 120/65 whereas a 60-year-old 140/80.

Blood glucose control

Where is your blood glucose now? A fasting blood glucose should be around 4 (UK) 70-99 mg/di (US). When your doctor or nurse takes an HbA1C level they are checking historic levels over a period of two to three months. A normal level for someone who is not diabetic would be below 42 mmol/mol (UK) 4-5.9% (US).

Body fat

The worrying fat we know about tends to be called visceral fat and that's the fat that can accumulate around your organs and can be dangerous to health.

Bone density

Your bones are porous bits of tissue and in women, they start to decline in your 30's. Bone density is a measure of your biological age and weight bearing-exercise, even when you are older, can increase bone density.

Cholesterol levels

You've maybe heard the expression good cholesterol and bad cholesterol. The point is the body produces cholesterol in the liver and it is used to produce bile, certain hormones and tissue building.

When you get your cholesterol measured it's good to be around 5 (UK) 200mg per deciliter or lower (US). You also want your HDL-high density lipoprotein level to be above 1 (UK) 60 mg/dl (US). Too high an LDL-low-density lipoprotein level could lead to hardening of the arteries and thus a stroke. (Some pharmacies offer private testing facilities if you are not being monitored by your doctor).

Hormone levels

You may have noticed that changes in your body, indicative of lower oestrogen and progesterone levels, have produced different effects - some quite distressing.

Immune function

How many infections have you had this year? Cold sores, styes, respiratory infections, to name but three show that you have a low immune function.

Metabolic activity

This is the activity that the body uses when converting food to energy and where possible weight gain can occur if this activity cannot deal adequately with increased calories.

Muscle mass and strength

When we look at telomere length then we know that certain types of exercise lengthen telomeres - an indication of biological age and I discuss that in the exercise section.

Skin thickness

As we age our skin becomes thinner. That equates to a longer healing time when skin is damaged, as mentioned above.

Temperature regulation

The ability of your body to deal with increases in temperature is a marker of your biological age.

Visual acuity

When did you start to need glasses for the first time - 40 or 50? Short-sightedness starts to set in because of ageing and although there are exercises that can help e.g. the Bates method[3] (his work has been generally discredited), replacement lens or laser therapy can sometimes restore 20/20 vision.

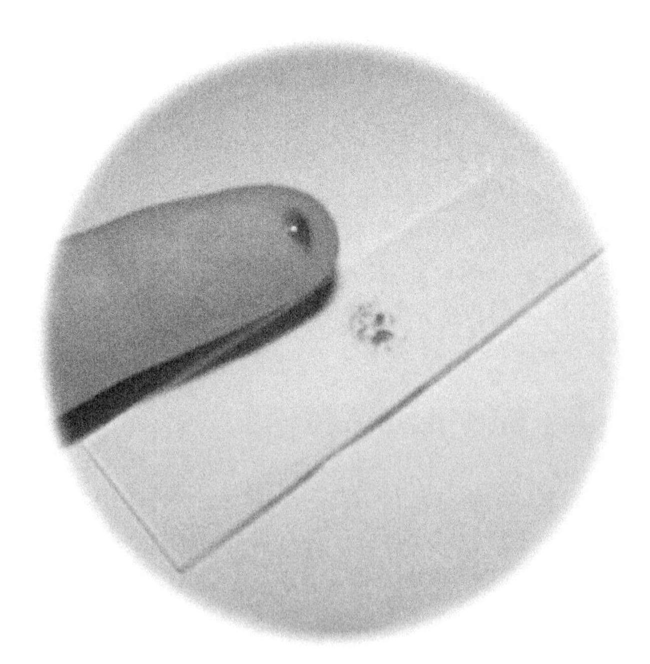

This section of the book has been about both the mental and physical aspects of ageing. I've shown some research, other anecdotal information, and I hope you have found something that you can do to improve the ageing process.

TIPS AND THOUGHTS

1. Are there things you can do to reduce your biological age?
2. Are there mental health aspects that need to be addressed?

Chapter 6

L is for Lifestyle

Do you think how you look is important? Do you feel a lift after going to the hairdressers, or does that not matter to you? During Covid-19, there wasn't a choice, with hairdressers shut. Then, many women came up with the suggestion that getting their hair 'done' was the number one priority when lockdown eased.

Many women put themselves through quite dramatic punishment to change the way they look.

Have you ever considered Botox, for instance? Botulinum toxin is injected into your face using a fine needle. It stops neurotransmitters from signalling muscles to contract, thus causing the relaxation of wrinkles. It is relatively safe provided the health professional is fully qualified and uses licensed preparations under strict risk assessments. The effect usually lasts between three and four months.

Putting a toxin into your body is, of course, your own decision and everyone has the choice to spend their money where they choose. Beautifying is absolutely fine, as long as it is your own choice and no one else's.

Drinking alcohol is another lifestyle choice, or is it? I have seen people being taunted or even forced to 'try' a drink as all around begin to feel the effects. Certainly, with the driving ban, it has been easier to refuse alcohol but drinking at home has somewhat become the norm during the restrictions.

So, what does alcohol do to your body? First of all, it is a poison but it also is known to give one a pleasant glow. When alcohol enters the body as well as crossing the blood-brain barrier, it has to be broken down by the liver before elimination. Crossing into the brain, it relaxes you but can also stimulate, so there are paradoxes of behaviour.

One person will be the life and soul of the party while another exhibiting almost depressive-like qualities. Metabolism leading to the elimination of alcohol requires water so it's a good idea to include that when you are having a drink.

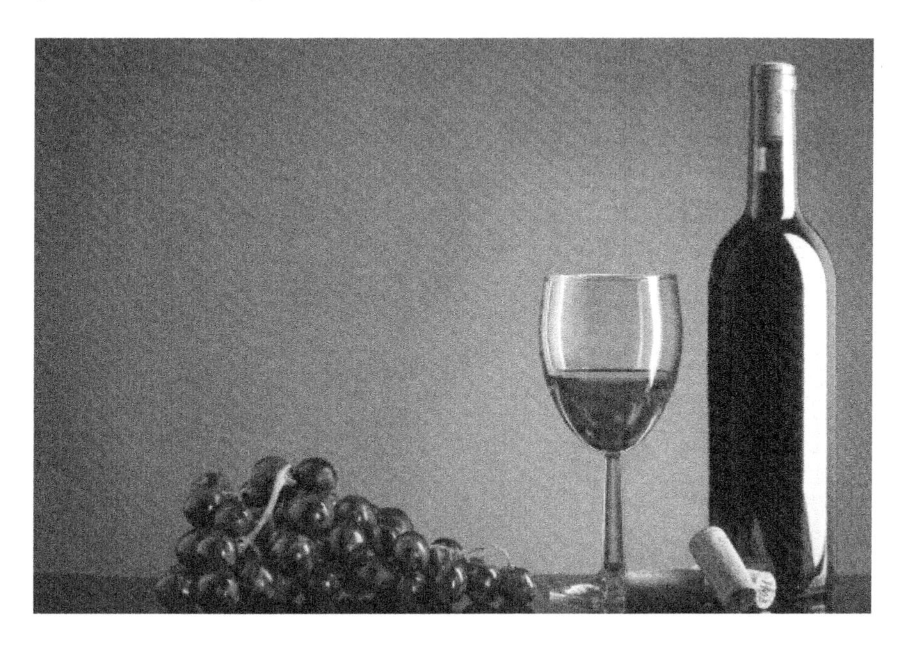

There are some good qualities of wine. Flavonoids are present in the skins of grapes. These have antioxidant qualities that can have beneficial effects on health. Some studies show a decrease in blood pressure but, like many things, the quantity of red wine needs to be moderate or any benefits will be lost.

What about sleep? Quality sleep is essential for giving you a quality life. You have probably experienced having one of those poor night's sleep where the next day you seem to be working well below par and just not feeling energised.

Modern lives do affect sleep. Simple points about the environment of the bedroom:

- Is it blacked out since that light coming in can stimulate the brain to wake up?
- The temperature needs to be about 16-18 degrees and all electrical equipment ideally should be removed from the bedroom.
- Blue light in particular affects the production of melatonin. That's the hormone produced by the pineal gland that promotes sleep.

Feng Shui is the ancient Chinese art of balancing two forces known as yin and yang so that the life force-qi-can be harmonised in the surroundings. Physically balancing your bedroom according to Feng Shui may be the answer to augmenting harmonisation.

Do you wind down for a while – ideally an hour before going to bed? With busy lives, you may forget the difference that turning off the television, having a warm bath and relaxing have on the quality of your sleep. It is worth thinking about.

What about the timing of your evening meal? The later you eat, particularly food that is high in fat content, requires greater digestion by your body and can interfere with the normal process. Caffeine from coffee and tea and even alcohol can affect sleep patterns. Yes, a small amount of alcohol, as already mentioned, can relax you but larger amounts can disrupt the sleep pattern and leave you tired in the morning. What you want to achieve is about 50% in a deep sleep. That is when your body repairs blood cells and tissues. The REM (Rapid Eye Movement) stage of sleep is when your brain is most active - you are dreaming. It is thought to be particularly important in your overall emotional well-being.

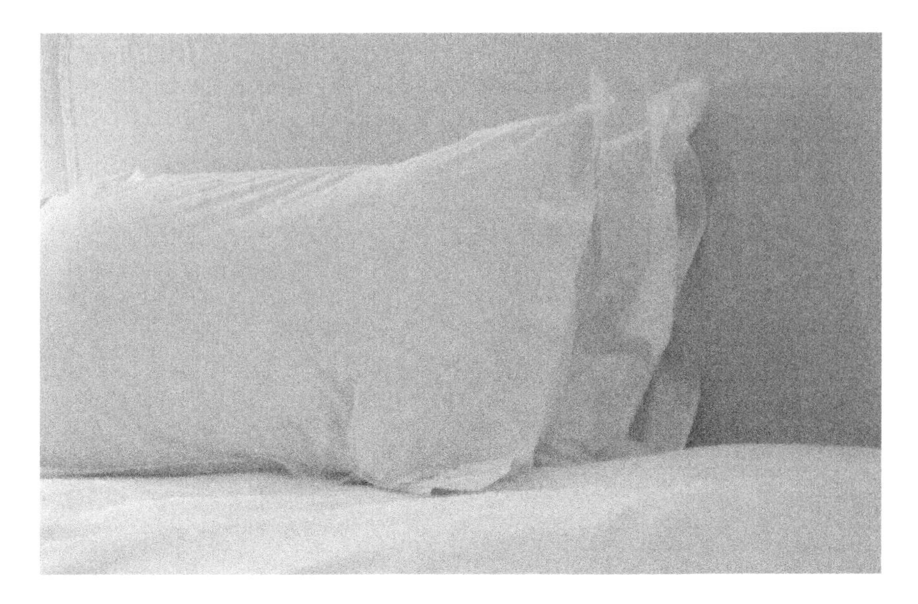

Debbie owned a high-class lingerie outlet in Edinburgh where she sold beautiful underwear, swimwear and night attire. There was a wonderful lightly perfumed smell when you entered her premises. Running this business did have its problems and Debbie was finding that more and more of her nights were being disrupted with episodes where she was wide awake - sometimes at four in the morning.

Debbie asked for advice and was looking at the environmental side of the bedroom environment. She tried, first of all, a simple remedy of putting a few drops of lavender on her pillow. 'But I smell the same as my grandmother', she complained but agreed to try it anyway.

She also wrote down all the things that she was going to have to attend to the next day as if it was already achieved. Such and such a bill was paid, x items had been ordered from a certain supplier and all her staff were in and had no problems as far as she understood. Gradually, with the ritual of eating earlier, preparing for bed with no electronics to stimulate her brain and writing down the next day's tasks as if they have been fulfilled, Jenny's sleep pattern improved.

She also got herself into the routine of going to bed and rising at the same times each day - even at weekends.

Quality sleep means you feel rested every day and able to get on with your tasks within a few minutes of rising.

What about diet concerning the quality of life? Hippocrates has said, "Food can be your medicine, and medicine can be your food."

I address food in chapter 10 - Longevity.

I deal with exercise in chapter 13 - another important component in making sure you achieve that quality of life.

THOUGHTS AND TIPS

1. Are there lifestyle issues you need to address?
2. Choose the important aspects for you to boost the quality of your life.

Chapter 7

I is for Irritations

I'm calling this chapter irritations rather than problems growing older, since I feel they can be addressed - sometimes with medication and sometimes with alternatives.

If I can start with the menopause. It is the change of life, and it is called that because there is a tremendous change in your hormone levels. When you were younger, you had your periods (usually every 28 days), but then they probably became less frequent, and that was because your ovaries were producing less oestrogen. There is a marked change in the amount and balance of the sex hormones.

This, as you know, produces a lot of effects: hot flushes, night sweats (sometimes during the day) and some psychological changes.

Juna was a high-flying executive. She had fought her way to the top, probably at the expense of family and friends, although she did not realise their importance until she suddenly noticed she was even starting to forget the important appointments. Panic started to set in. She would be sitting at a board meeting whilst feeling this tremendous heat starting around her chest and travelling up to her face, and coupled with embarrassment, she was struggling to find everyday words. 'I need to see my GP urgently', she thought – 'maybe it is the start of Alzheimer's?'

The appointment with the GP was set for the following Thursday. After some tests, the GP stated to an anxious Juna, 'No, I can assure you it is not the start of dementia and Alzheimers as you were fearing, it is simply the menopause.'

Juna's body started to relax, and then she began asking questions. 'What can I do about it?' 'Well', Dr Shukaf explained 'there are a few things we can do medically if you like? HRT – that's hormone replacement therapy.'

'Does that not bring risks?' asked Juna.

'Yes', the doctor answered 'but you've got to look at them in proportion. First of all, there is a small increase in the risk of cancer with oral HRT and it is related to how long you stay on the medicine. Is that something you would like to try?'

Juna thought for a minute about what her life had been like in the last few weeks.

'Yes, I need to try it to help bring my body back to equilibrium again'.

So, Juna left the surgery with her prescription and headed to the pharmacy so that she could start the medication as quickly as possible.

Yes, it did make a dramatic difference but Juna realised the older she got the greater are the risks of taking the medication.

There are also benefits such as reducing the risk of osteoporosis. Osteoporosis is a condition that weakens bones. They become more fragile, and you are more likely to have a break. HRT reduces long term risk for around 10 years. Taking the medicine also has a beneficial effect on the risk of heart attacks. The Nurses Health Study in America showed the risk of a heart attack can be reduced by 50%.

There are alternatives to oestrogen. Progestogens, such as tibolone, in high doses can help with menopausal symptoms. It acts similarly to some HRT products but doesn't seem to have the same risk on breast cancer incidence.

Progesterone creams have not shown benefit in relieving symptoms, but how does a prescriber decide which product is right for you?

He or she must decide on the reason for prescribing a particular dose. Is it for prevention or reversal of adverse symptoms? It has got to be adequate, but at the same time low enough to avoid side effects, if possible.

A woman who has had a hysterectomy will only need oestrogen, whereas women with an intact womb will take a combination of progesterone and oestrogen.

If bone protection is required, for those diagnosed with osteoporosis, then bisphosphonates are prescribed. These sometimes have been shown to have problems with administration. Alendronic acid, for example, a weekly medicine must be taken at least half an hour before food or other medication. You must be standing or sitting upright, and the tablet is taken with a full glass of water. Apart from the side effects, inflammation of the oesophagus (the tube leading from the mouth to the stomach), if the tablets are not taken correctly, there is a small incidence of necrosis of the jaw. Because of the potential effect of the medicine on bone in the jaw, it's important to have a check-up with your dentist regarding taking the medication. You should always have a review after 5 years of taking it.

Alternatives from hormone preparations are products

like plant-based remedies. Substances such as Red Clover contain phytoestrogens - plant oestrogens. Some of the evidence suggests relief from hot flushes and night sweats but they don't protect you from the long-term oestrogen deficiency disease. We also do not know if there are any long-term adverse effects but, the fact they have been used for years, suggests a reasonable safety/efficacy ratio. Omega 3 (as mentioned in chapter 12 Fats) has been shown to relieve hot flushes and as there are many benefits from taking this particular fat, I suggest it is worth trying. The next two 'irritations' as I like to call them are vaginal dryness and incontinence.

Sally realised that sex was becoming painful. She knew if she did not do something about it soon, her marriage was going to falter. She had never been fully able to discuss their sexual relationship, so she decided the best thing to do was to go to her doctor and ask if there was anything she could get on a prescription.

Dr Sanches, thankfully, was very understanding and made Sally feel at ease when she visited him at the surgery. 'I am going to give you a cream which you apply internally. You use it every night for 2-3 weeks, then twice weekly, and I would like to see you in 2 months where we may stop the treatment and then assess whether we need to start up again. There is, of course, possible side effect - hyperplasia (an overproduction of cells).

'Thanks, doctor', said Sally and as she headed home after picking up the cream from the pharmacy, she knew she would have to have that conversation with Alan, her husband. Instead of it being a difficult conversation, Alan was completely understanding and after a few weeks they were enjoying their sexual activity once again. There is some research to suggest that flooding your body with hormones during orgasm has an anti-ageing benefit, as well as providing pleasure.

The 'topical' oestrogen preparations come in a cream form as described but also as pessaries that are inserted into the vagina. Some women get a vaginal ring for a prolapse of the womb and this is fitted by a nurse but all of these should be discussed with your doctor so that you find the correct one for you. There are also non-hormonal lubricants. Most pharmacies will have an array of lubricants on their shelves. Your doctor can also prescribe some e.g. Replens and Yes (in the UK). If sorting this 'irritation' out means you have a better quality of life, then don't hesitate to find out what is right for you.

Another 'irritation' that I have referred to above is incontinence - there are four types. The first is 'stress' incontinence when you cough, sneeze or exercise and your bladder is under pressure. The second is urge incontinence when urine leaks when you have a strong desire to empty your bladder. The third is overflow incontinence, which is also called chronic urinary retention, which means you can't fully empty your bladder and that can lead to leaks. The final type is total incontinence when you have lost control of your bladder - it can't store urine, so you have frequent leaking. So, what are the causes of this difficult 'irritation?'

In stress incontinence, your pelvic floor muscles or the muscle around your urethra could be weak or damaged so that you are unable to retain the urine. You could have damaged these muscles through childbirth or being chronically obese. If you have had certain types of surgery such as a hysterectomy or are suffering from Parkinson's disease or Multiple Sclerosis, then these conditions can lead to incontinence.

Urge incontinence is generally a result of a weakening of the detrusor muscles in your bladder. These muscles relax and contract when the bladder is filling and when you are voiding urine. If these muscles contract too often the brain then creates an urgency to pass urine. It could be too much caffeine or alcohol but conversely, if the urine becomes too concentrated through dehydration, then this can irritate and sensitise the bladder wall thus causing the problem. If you are constipated, then that can result in a strain on muscles with extra leakage.

Overflow incontinence can be because there is an obstruction. In that case, you will not be able to completely empty the bladder and, of course, this can cause urine to leak out. Constipation once again can be a cause or if you have had an operation that has affected nerves in the area.

Total incontinence is where the bladder is incapable of storing urine and you have no control. This could have been caused by a birth defect or injury to your spinal cord. There is also a condition where there is a physical 'tunnel' formed between the vagina and the bladder.

Of course, some medicines cause incontinence - diuretics - they are used for removing excess fluid from the body through the bladder. You may be on an ACE (angiotensin-converting enzyme) inhibitor for blood pressure or heart failure or are taking sedatives or antidepressants.

Now that I have shown you the different types of incontinence - what can you do about it if you are suffering?

Obviously, the type of incontinence will require a different regime but generally, lifestyle changes are a good place to start.

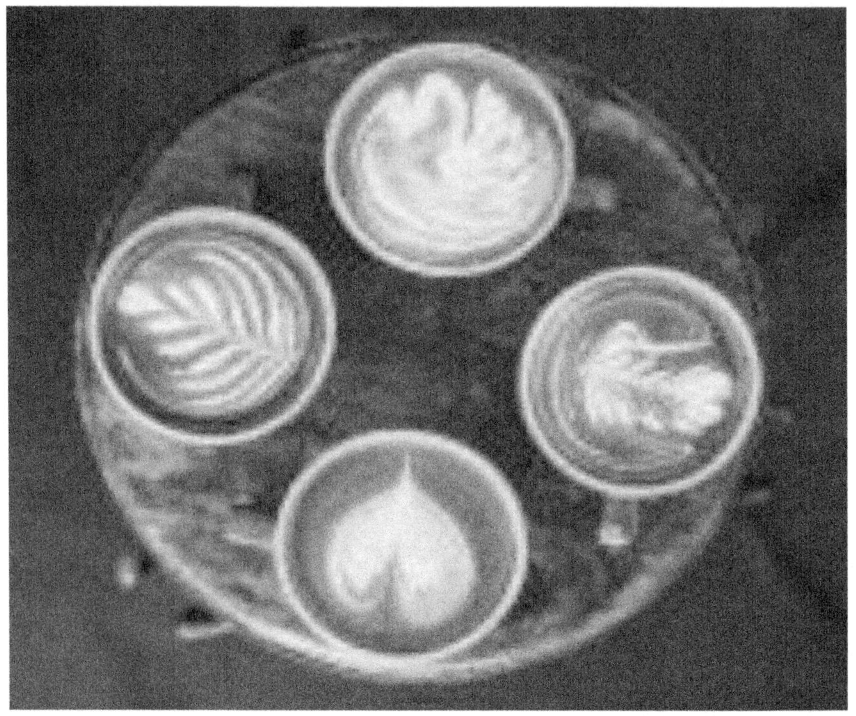

How much coffee do you drink? Is that causing a problem? As I have said previously, drinking too much or too little can affect your urine output. Try and have a happy medium regarding fluid intake, and that may settle things. It is an individual thing, so experiment until you find success.

What about your weight? You can find out your BMI (body mass index) by calculating weight against height, including your age on a BMI calculator. You want to be somewhere between 20 and 25. Being in that weight range will help reduce incontinence. (There is a move away from BMI measurement to waist size. A woman around 50 ideally should have a waist size of less than 35 inches).

One of the mainstays of improving continence particularly for stress incontinence is strengthening the pelvic floor muscles. These muscles surround the urethra and the bladder and are responsible for controlling the flow of urine.

Discovering where your pelvic floor muscles are can prove problematic. The best way to describe them is when you void urine if you stop the flow then that is your stimulating the correct muscles.

It is best to find an expert in pelvic floor exercises who can teach you the correct method. The NHS (in the UK) offers continence services in your area. They are normally provided by a team of continence nurses who assess your position and can advise on whether it is the physical use of pads or other treatments that are required. You usually access these services through your GP. Physiotherapists with expertise in incontinence is also a route to go down where you will be taught by an expert on how to perform the exercises. Normally, it includes a minimum of 8 muscle contractions at least 3 times a day and lasts for at least 3 months.

Doing exercises at home may help. Squeezing the muscles around your vagina and anus as if you were holding in the urine is exercising the pelvic floor.

Try and not to hold your breath or tense the muscles in your buttocks when you do the exercise. Build up the length of time you hold the contraction - count to 20.

12 weeks is an approximate time needed to notice a difference and, of course, continuing with the exercises is important afterwards as well.

Usually, with an expert, there are bladder training exercises where you train your bladder to resist the urge to urinate. The idea is that you increase the time between voiding and hopefully regain control so there is reduced rushing to the toilet.

There is also electrical stimulation of the muscles. There are companies that advise the wearing of garments for 30 minutes five times a week and there is also direct stimulation in the vagina with a probe that artificially exercises the muscles. (This can sometimes be unpleasant).

Vaginal cones that are inserted inside are available. Each cone, as you progress, is a heavier weight.

Finally, there are incontinence pads and garments. The companies realise that potentially this is a huge and growing market and have now designed sheer, unobtrusive products of all shapes and sizes. Remember these products are designed for urine and are quite different from sanitary products. They are made so that they can contain in some cases quite large volumes of urine without leakage and also deodorise so that you can feel confident that no one will notice.

So, what about medicine for stress incontinence?

There are various medicines on the market. Each has

a benefit but also some side effects. There is a range of medicines called antimuscarinics. Examples are oxybutynin and tolterodine that are for an overactive bladder. They work well but side effects include constipation, dry mouth, blurred vision, tiredness and in some cases a buildup of pressure in the eye - glaucoma.

For stress incontinence, there is a medicine called duloxetine. It increases the muscle tone of the urethra. (The tube that carries urine outside the body). Its side effects are similar to antimuscarinics, but you are better not stopping the medicine abruptly. Talk to your doctor first.

There is an alternative medicine available called mirabegron. It allows the muscle to relax and therefore the bladder to fill up. Side effects include a propensity to infections in the urinary tract, heartbeat irregularity and itchy skin. Like all of these medicines there is a balancing act between helping you with the condition, but at the same time minimising any side effects.

In extreme cases, your doctor may prescribe catheters (tubes that are fitted into the urethra) that in some women can change lives.

There is a final medicine that is useful for nighttime frequency - desmopressin. It reduces the amount of urine produced so you don't need to get up so often during the night time.

The other 'nuisance' I would like to talk about is where you are worried that your memory is beginning to go. I realise that dementia possibly leading to Alzheimer's is not something we have managed to find a cure for to date (2021), but there are techniques that can improve your memory that are worth trying.

Turn off the television. We know that stimulation from an increased amount of viewing is really not exercising your brain in a meaningful way.

Have you ever been standing with a friend and you see someone coming towards you who you know very well, and you know you will have to introduce them to your friend, but you can't remember their name?

Dominic O'Brien is a world memory champion whose memory improves every year - how does that happen? Many of us think our memory is declining. Is it possible to improve it?

The said gentleman, as an after-dinner speaker, enthrals his audience by his memory triumphs. Say there are 100 people at the dinner and each table has a host plus 9 guests. At the beginning of the evening, Dominic would approach each table and ask the host to introduce him to each guest. He would then eat his meal and after coffee be introduced as the speaker of the evening 'World Memory Champion Dominic O'Brien'. He would then stand up and starting with table one he would go round the table stating each person's name until he had mentioned the 100 guests. Everyone is, of course, always astonished. He then explains how he does it. 'It's association, location and imagination.'

When you meet someone for the first time say their name as you shake hands and look at their face. Does this person remind you of someone? Maybe your cousin. In order to remember the person's name, you need to put the familiar face in a location that will remind you of that person i.e. put the face in your cousin's garden.

Say the person is called Daisy. Then you put 'Daisy' in your cousin's garden. Now the imagination comes into play. You see in your imagination standing on a 'Munro' – that's the name of mountains in Scotland - but you also see your cousin covered in daisies and standing on a Munro. Yes, the name of this lady is Daisy Munro.

You can have lots of fun with this. How about you meet someone who looks like a doctor. Say his name is George so you transport this person to your surgery, and you imagine a George who is famous - George Clooney, for example. Now the person's second name is Baker, so you see someone who looks like George Clooney sitting in your doctor's surgery with a baker's hat on.

Another technique is making mental images regarding a person's name. Pat Whitehead could be depicted in your memory as seeing your enormous hand dripping with white paint patting the top of her head.

You can remember people's names if you practice, but that obviously requires you to do the work. Are you going to try?

But what about stimulating parts of your brain that are not used to it? Have you tried writing with your left hand? It probably starts off with a childlike scrawl but as you improve you will begin to write legibly and at the same time stimulate new areas in the brain. There are those who have spent their lives being good at say figures e.g. accountants or mathematicians. What I suggest you do if you are in that category then learn to dance - that is right - again use different parts of your brain. It will also be a form of relaxation away from an intense book or computer work.

Learning a language is known to improve the brain. MRI scans of the brain can show stimulation in certain areas - the hippocampus and cerebral cortex known to be responsible for memory.

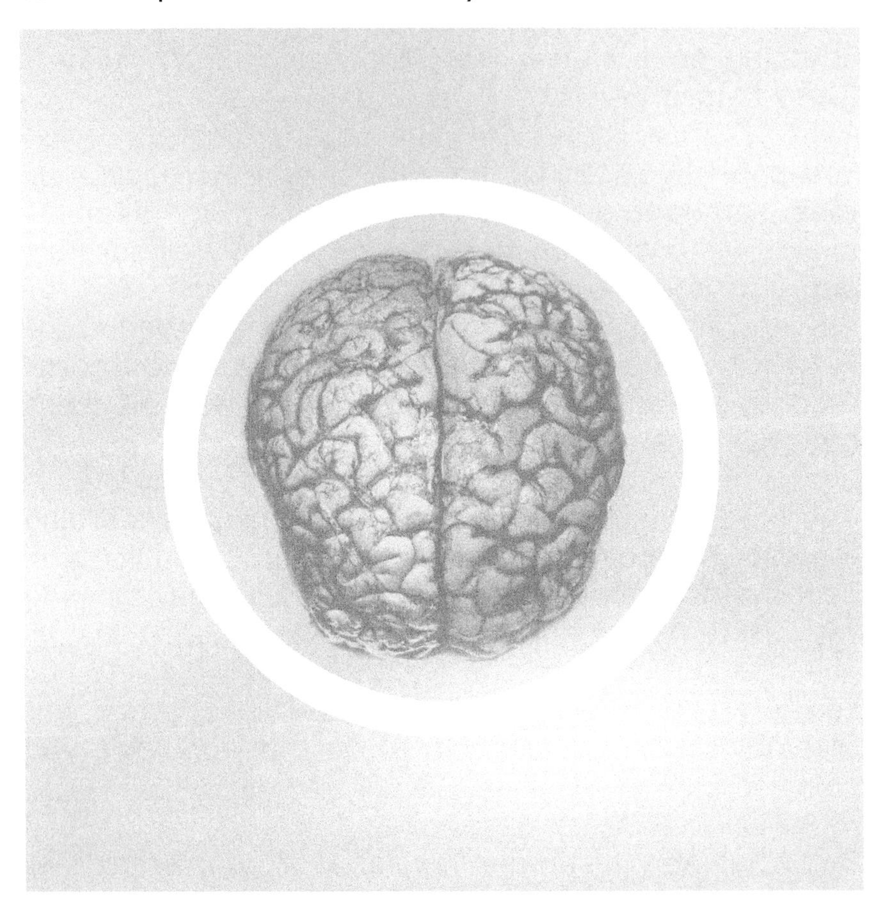

Lastly 'my hair is falling out - what can I do?'

If someone approaches me with that issue the first thing, I say to them 'get a blood test at your doctor's practice'. What they will be looking for is an imbalance relating to your thyroid gland or a low iron level. If either of these problems are found, then the good news is they can be remedied with medication. Severe stress can also cause premature hair loss.

There is also something called Minoxidil. It was originally developed for high blood pressure but one of the side effects was hair growth. It comes in a preparation that you rub on the scalp. Of course, as soon as you stop applying the lotion hair growth stops so it's a lifestyle choice.

We have not got all the answers to the irritations in growing older, but we can address some of the issues to improve the quality of your life.

TIPS AND THOUGHTS

1. Address any physical issues with your GP or through your own research.
2. Think about how you can stimulate the brain. Do something different in your life.

chapter 8

T is for alTernatives

Sometimes it is useful to look at alternatives, maybe for a physical problem or an emotional one. (See section on EFT chapter 18).

Homoeopathy does not fare well as a subject with scientists. There are three principles concerning homoeopathy. The first is the Law of Similars that means administering a substance to effect a cure renders similar symptoms in a healthy individual. (That means with aggravation the problem can get worse before getting better).

The second principle is the use of the infinitesimal dose to restore health. This principle is so that the least harm is exerted on the patient. It is all about dilution but also succussion - vigorous shaking as the therapeutic qualities are secured. In homoeopathy, the more dilution and succussion that takes place the greater the increase in healing power. (This seems contradictory to allopathic or ordinary medicine).

It is the theory that once the product has been diluted 24 times there is, in fact, no original molecule. Therefore, that is why it is hard for a scientist to believe there could be any therapeutic or healing effect.

The third principle, which I think is probably the most important, is the holistic approach to treating an individual. This principle is one that I wholeheartedly agree with since a practitioner should treat the 'whole' person not just the disease itself.

When you attend a homoeopathic practitioner, they illicit a complete picture of you including your temperament. It is important for you to work yourself, particularly balancing issues in your life, quality of your sleep and excesses (see Chapter 6 Lifestyle), or Exercise (chapter 13). The environmental and social aspects of your life are all taken into consideration when choosing a remedy.

I also mentioned temperament. One preparation will work with one individual and not another. Choosing the correct remedy for you takes time - an appointment with a homoeopath may be over an hour but I also think taking time with any practitioner who listens wholly to you is a kind of healing on its own.

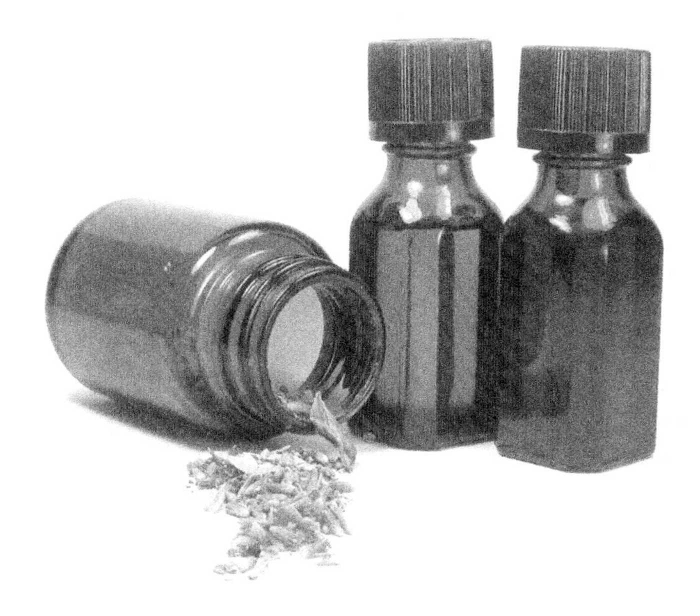

And when you are given a remedy, it is important to handle it properly. I say handle it properly since that is the first rule. It should not be put in your hand where it could be contaminated by soap or nowadays alcoholic sanitisers.

It should be kept away from light, mobile phones and strong perfumes. It is also important to take the remedy in a clean mouth. That means 15 minutes on either side of eating, drinking or cleaning your teeth. Incidentally, caffeine is something you should try and avoid for the duration of the treatment since it has an adverse effect on the healing effect of the remedy.

If you are thinking of trying homoeopathy, then I suggest you seek out a qualified homoeopath. Buying a remedy off the shelf rarely works.

Is it possible to 'cure' something like labyrinthitis with alternatives - in this case, particular exercises?

Labyrinthitis is related to a sensitivity in the balance mechanism in the inner ear. Have you ever felt really drunk - surely not - or maybe felt quite sick on a boat? What is happening is that your brain is disconnecting with your physical surroundings and you feel sick and might even vomit.

Some people live with this condition all their lives. It could be brought on initially from a viral infection but sometimes excess stress and generally ant-emetics-anti sickness tablets are prescribed to settle things down.

As an alternative, there are vestibular exercises. These exercises create feelings of dizziness but eventually they disappear. You must not ever do the exercises if you have a headache, and they need to be done after an appointment with a vestibular expert – a Chartered Physiotherapist specialising in Vestibular Conditions and Rehabilitation (i.e. dizziness and balance issues). (See the back of the book for a recommendation).

I heard that the late Bruce Forsyth had practised vestibular exercises for years and I don't know if you noticed on 'Strictly' his balance was quite extraordinary for his age.

Cannabinoids (CBD) in oil, tincture and capsule form are now creating a bit of a stir as being useful for all sorts of problems, from anxiety to pain and even epilepsy. I should say at the start that the medicinal products that are starting to be licensed for therapeutic use such as epilepsy are not the same as the products you buy over the counter. There is an element in cannabis – THC – that gives the known effects on the brain - the highs and mood changing mechanisms. This part of the cannabinoids that are available contain only a tiny percentage of that element yet have, in some cases, quite remarkable effects. The analgesic or painkilling effect is now well known and I have patients who use less of their ordinary pain-killing tablets as a result of taking these products. People also tell me that they have found they are much more relaxed when taking cannabinoid preparations.

Herbal medicines are quite different from homoeopathic preparations. Interestingly, many of our modern drugs have evolved from herbal substances. Willow bark, for example, has been used in the past as a pain reliever. The active ingredient in the medicine made from willow bark is called salicin. Aspirin is acetylsalicylic acid – the synthetic form of the product and as well as bringing down a high temperature we are finding new uses such as prevention of colon cancer. St John's wort is a herb for use in low mood and anxiety. It is important to use the product according to the manufacturer's instructions and be aware of interactions with other medicines.

Another herb such as Ginkgo Biloba has been used traditionally to reduce memory loss and enhance circulation. There can be side effects with this such as nausea, diarrhoea and headache. Interactions with traditional medicines are common with this herb so best to check with your doctor or pharmacist if you are thinking of trying it out.

It is important to realise that herbal medicines could affect the absorption of some allopathic medicines or may enhance their effect in the body e.g. Ginkgo with blood-thinning medicines. This is unlike the homoeopathic medicines that can be taken with but not at exactly the same time, as medication on prescription.

Reiki is another alternative healing process. Its meaning from Japanese is 'spiritually guided life force energy.' A reiki master is able to stimulate parts of the body by laying on of hands to discover blockages in the flow of energy that could be causing health issues. Negative thoughts and feelings can contribute to illness and reiki seek to calm negativity so that natural healing can take place.

Tara had what she thought was an insurmountable problem. Rashes were appearing in odd places on her body, and she seemed to have exhausted all the normal treatments - antifungal creams, moisturisers and steroids. She was advised to change her washing powder and keep a diary of things she was eating. She also threw out her normal skin preparations and changed to herbal products to see if that made a difference.

As nothing had seemed to work, she decided to go down the alternative route.

The importance of alternatives is once again looking at the whole person. What was going on in her life? Was she under a lot of stress? The answers to these questions were 'yes'. She had family problems on top of trying to hold down a full-time job.

She had read about reiki but had limited knowledge of it. It just seemed it was 'worth a try.' The reiki sessions allowed Tara to focus on herself and, of course, she began to realise that she was self-sabotaging. Her health was taking a back seat while she engaged in this stressful lifestyle. By slowing down this energy and realigning with healthy meridians Tara calmed down and her rashes started to disappear.

Is this something you can relate to?

Another alternative that has been used through the ages is hypnosis. Hypnosis got a bad name during the '70s and '80s since practitioners would use stage shows to show people in compromising positions, for example pretending to be a hen clucking across the stage when in a hypnotic trance.

Nowadays hypnosis is used even in medical situations, for example dentistry, to relax a patient before treatment.

When you are in a hypnotic state your brain waves ideally should be in the range 7hz to 8hz - that is between alpha and theta. Your brain should be able to promote the thoughts that are being fed into you by the hypnotist while still being conscious of what is happening to you, for example your environment, and if there was any danger you would react but at the same time, you would be in a deeply relaxed state.

Using this type of intervention quite dramatic changes can be made - weight loss, giving up smoking, sorting outlasting harmful images from the past.

Kirsten had a throat problem. Ever since she had had a viral infection, it had caused her to cough and clear her throat for many weeks. In desperation, she decided to consult a hypnotist to try and resolve the issue and he started to talk to her about her life. She was in a caring profession and took responsibility for the people in her remit.

The problem was as she talked about it, her over caring attitude was making her ill and she realised that no one was particularly caring for her.

The hypnotist expertly guided Kirsten first of all into a relaxed state and then asked her to imagine walking in the countryside and on her left was a black stallion galloping around the field completely free and untethered. He asked her if she could imagine that feeling herself of being relaxed and happy. It did take three treatments for Kirsten to address her health issue by adjusting her life, but it did work.

The last alternative I am going to write about is acupuncture. Like many of the ancient Chinese healing practices, it relies on stimulating certain points on the body along channels or meridians. Some people compare these meridians with the circulatory system, but they involve energy as opposed to plasma. Each of the meridians has a specific number and acupuncture points relating to parts of the body.
Meridians are like a network. However, meridians are not visible, but rather energetic. Each of the 14 meridian channels has a specific number, and acupuncture points all have meanings.

In the western world, acupuncture has now been recognised as a treatment for pain.

Nice Guidelines (UK) (these are guidelines drawn up by experts looking at the evidence) recommend a course of treatment for patients but only if it is delivered in a community setting, delivered by a band 7 or lower healthcare professional, and is made up of no more than 5 hours of healthcare professional time.

A Tens machine - that stands for transcutaneous electrical nerve stimulation - is a method of pain relief involving the use of a mild electrical current. The machine is a small, battery-operated device that sends the charge down leads to pads. These pads are placed on particular points on the body. Used properly, they can be used to stimulate meridians and cause pain relief to take place. Tens machines can be purchased online or from a pharmacy.

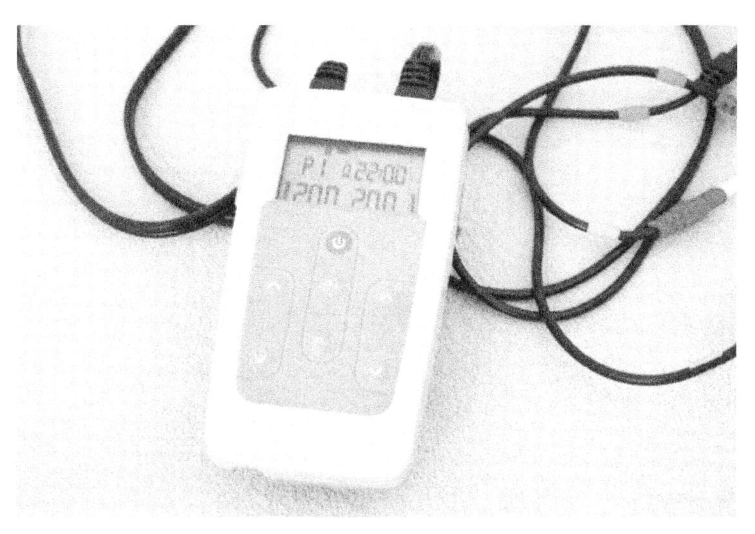

This section demonstrates just some of the alternatives available to deal with a variety of issues. Sometimes you don't realise you have an issue that is causing the problem, and that's why I have included some ideas at this stage in the book.

TIPS AND THOUGHTS

1. Did you find something that resonates with you?
2. Are you willing to try out an alternative for a specific problem?

Chapter 9

Y is for You

This chapter is about YOU. Often women do not think about themselves first and that can lead to health issues manifesting themselves or even a lack of fulfilment.

Cara was someone that seemed to lack confidence. She came to see me about a health matter but like many women, I could see she was lacking in self-esteem. I knew that that had to be addressed first before real healing could take place. I decided, with her permission, to use Neuro-Linguistic Programming or NLP.

NLP was developed in the 1970s by John Grinder (Linguistic Professor from the University of California, U.S.) who, working with Richard Bandler and Frank Pucelik, studied human excellence. Working to teaching psychotherapy, they were able to demonstrate healing and fulfilment.

Having attended training on NLP and 'graduated' as an NLP Master Practitioner I have used this skill to help patients throughout the years. It involves talking therapy, some parts of which have been morphed into Cognitive Behavioural Therapy (CBT), and used within the NHS to treat a wide variety of health issues. It is also used to help NHS staff to cope with work-related stress.

But to go back to Cara I decided, using questioning techniques, to start to discover what had happened in her life in the past to try and find a trigger where, once that is released, everything falls into place and healing can take place.

'It was at school' she said 'the girls would make fun of my leg that was slightly shorter than the other. It meant I had an irregular gait and that made me very self-conscious'.

With that information I was then able to use a light trance, to go back in time to when these mocking incidents took place. Cara was guided so that in her mind her classmates would crowd around her not to make fun of her but to praise her and want to be her friend. In the scenario created she was the most popular girl in the school.

This mental training had to be repeated but over two sessions I could see from Cara's face that she had changed. Her demeanour meant she visibly grew since she was no longer cowering down, eyes on the ground. About one week later Cara's husband arrived and said 'I am not sure what you did with Cara, but I just wanted to shake your hand and thank you.' NLP can work in certain circumstances, but each individual has to be assessed as to whether that is the best route.

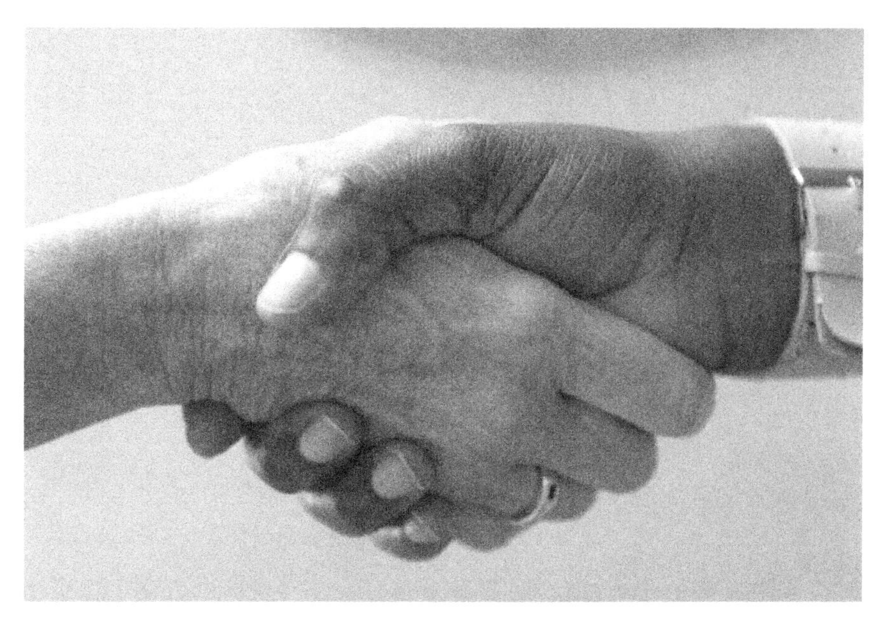

Sylvia had just retired and wanted to start an online course to help women who were suffering from stress and anxiety in particular. The first thing she did was train as a Cognitive Behavioural Therapist. She then offered her services post-COVID, where mental health issues had virtually exploded. Yes, she was now living her dream with a huge amount of satisfaction.

Do you take time for yourself?

A process that I find very helpful can be as short as six minutes. Can you give yourself 6 minutes? I am talking about the process of Mindfulness. It is being in the present and allowing your mind to just 'be' as opposed to being constantly active. The best way to learn Mindfulness is to take part in a group session. I, myself, have benefited from this. Being very stressed at work, I found I was not relaxing sufficiently at home. Listening to a Mindfulness CD (having learnt the technique in class) meant I was able to enjoy my leisure time in a much healthier way.

<u>TIPS AND THOUGHTS</u>

1. Can you relate to any of the issues in this chapter?
2. Could you give yourself 'me' time to recharge your battery?

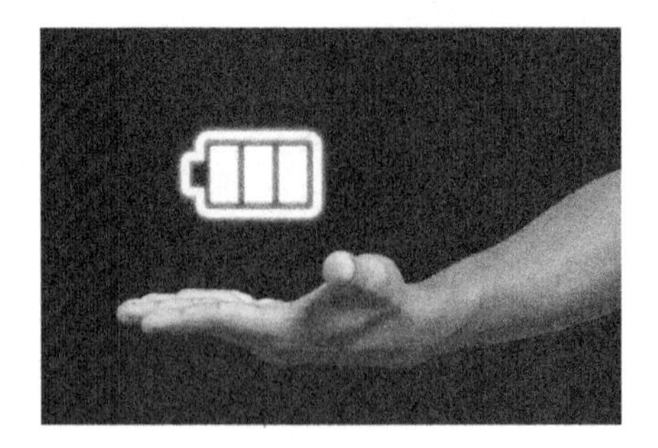

Chapter 10

L is for Longetivity

Do you want to live a long life? This book is all about quality, not so much the length of life. Let us look first of all at peoples around the world who seem to have both.

The Hunzas live in Hunza Valley in Pakistan. They live up to the ages of 120 or 140 but interestingly, death comes not from heart disease or cancer but old age. (This will inevitably mean that their heart stops but not - as I say from disease - it just 'wears out'). They can be seen playing sport in their 90's, and it is not uncommon for them to be fathering a child in their 80's and beyond. One of the main reasons for this long, healthy life is the predominance of unprocessed food in their diets. Another is the absolute respect the elders in the community are given by younger members. Psychologically this gives the elders strength, dignity and purpose in life.

I do not particularly address diet in other chapters, so I will do so here. In the supplement section, I suggest that the western diet is lacking in many nutrients - thus the need to take vitamins and minerals as well. If we look at the micronutrients in raw foods, these are the enzymes, minerals and vitamins that are vital for health, we end up destroying much of the nutrient value as we process them - heat, fry, barbecue.

Vitamin C, for example, loses its potency by about 10% per day. Imagine an orange coming from Spain, then being stored in a warehouse, before appearing on supermarket shelves. By the time you buy the orange, take it home and eat it, 7-10 days could have passed. The fibrous makeup of the orange is still, of course, beneficial but the vitamin C content will have reduced greatly.

Diet is an important component of health in old age, and having a percentage of raw food will enhance that benefit. Fat and sugar is a common combination in western diets. The problem is it makes us fat and sluggish, but yes, I know it tastes good. An example of an energy-sapping meal is Eid, Thanksgiving or Christmas time, where, even though you are full, you still manage that last Belgian chocolate. Falling asleep in front of the television is proof that your body is trying to metabolise the food resulting in a desire to sleep, rather than give you energy.

The number of calories seems to play a part. Those who live long, healthy lives do not eat in excess. It has also been shown that periods of fasting can improve health. Mice with restricted calorie intake live longer than their compatriots fed increased amounts. Health parameters measured showed better outcomes in the calorie-controlled cohort.

Is there a woman out there that does not enjoy chocolate? The chocolate that is beneficial for your health needs to contain a reasonable percentage of cocoa solids - the antioxidant element of the product. And again, quantity plays a part - too much sugar and fat will nullify the benefit.

There have been lots of longevity studies, and one that stands out is the Nun's Study. Dr David Snowdon, an epidemiologist at the University of Kentucky, studied this group of nuns in the USA. Early life higher education was a factor in the lower incidence of Alzheimer's, but one of the main findings was that they remained busy teaching, working in the garden and exercising well into their 90's.

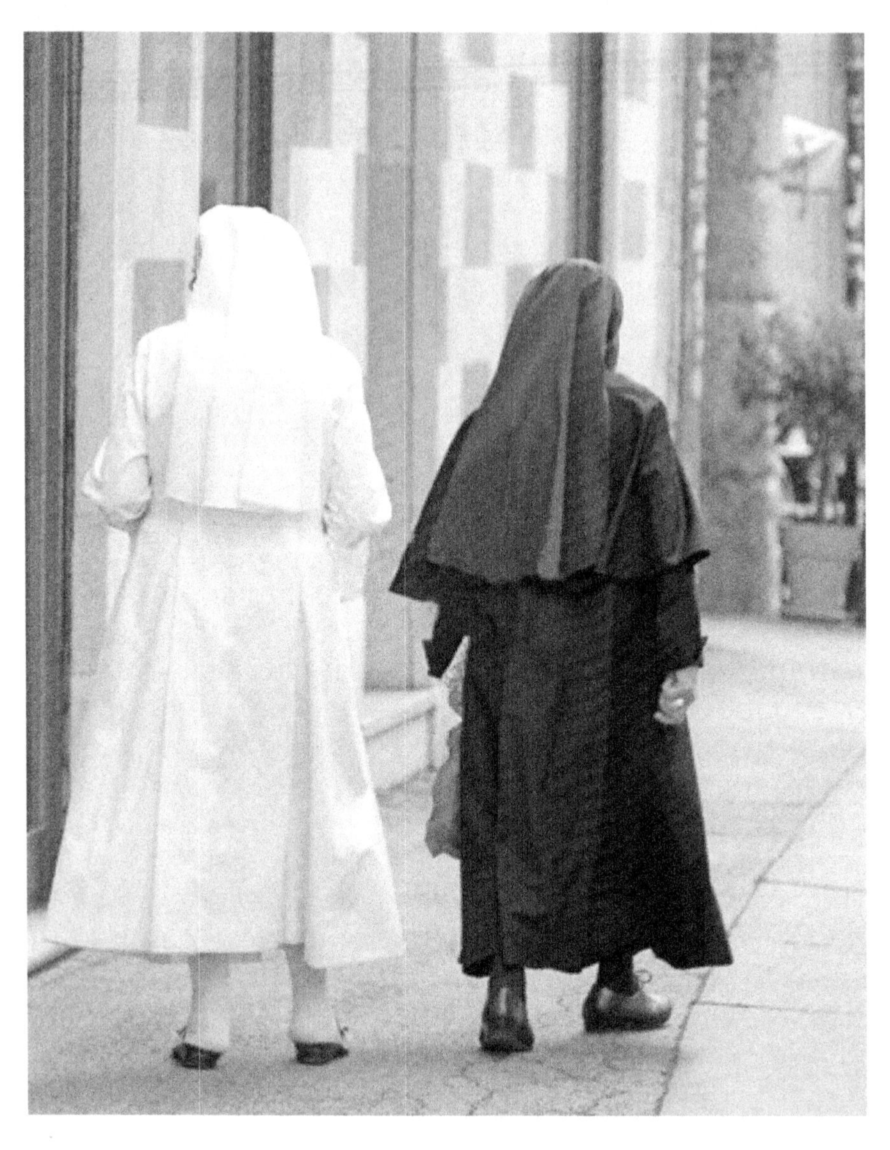

Having a purpose in life can give you a zest for living that is quite uncanny. Doing a job that is also your hobby can be uplifting. 'I am the luckiest person in the world,' said Mary. 'I'm in a caring role looking after an elderly lady, and it just brings me so much fulfilment that I don't feel I'm going to work every day.'

Professional work, where you find a great deal of satisfaction or doing tremendous work for a charity, can give you the boost you need – living your purpose. Have you found your purpose in life? Maybe having your family and letting them go, off to find their way, has been your purpose but have a look at Chapter 9 on 'You'. Maybe this is the time when new avenues open up, and your life takes a different direction - an exciting one.

Learning new techniques to boost your brain can help with the ageing process. I do not know if you have heard of 'Image Streaming'? I first heard about this when I was listening to a CD by Dr Win Wenger. Image streaming involves closing your eyes and imagining a scene. You then describe the scene out loud in the utmost detail - this is important - preferably with a partner, but even recording it can be effective. What is remarkable is that you will be able to remember the scene maybe even years later.

Another technique you may want to try is affirmations. You might have a voice inside your head that is sabotaging you. By that, I mean putting you down or constantly telling you something is not right, or you cannot do something?

What if you were to change that voice to 'I can do.... or I believe that I am.... ', and then finish with a positive statement?

It is best to do affirmations out loud, but I realise family members might not be on board, but this is for your benefit.

THOUGHTS AND TIPS

1. Try a new technique and see if that makes a difference.
2. Look at your diet and make sure you are giving your body all the nutrition it needs.

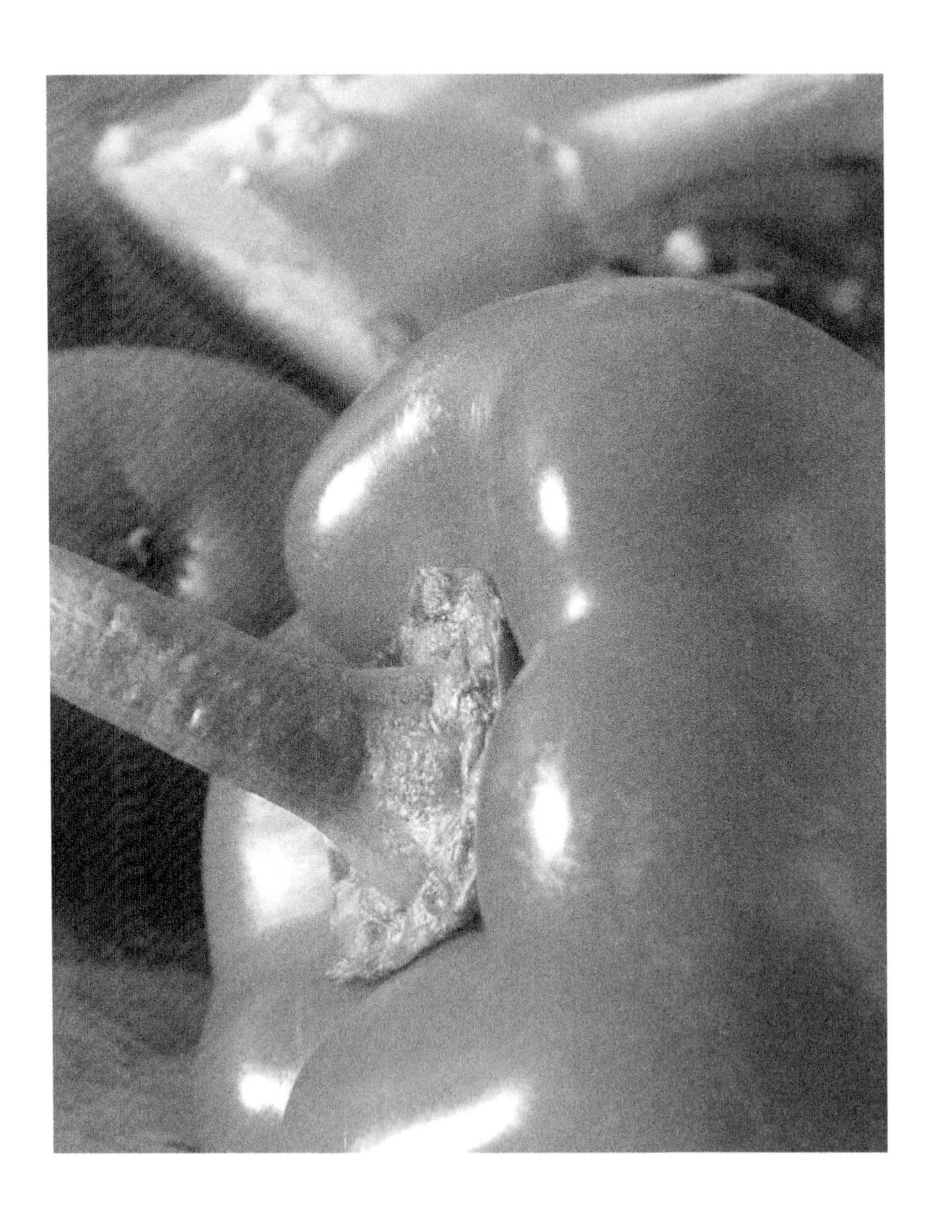

Chapter 11

I is for Inspiration

To be inspired is to be influenced. Maybe this thing or person has changed your life. I'm not going to dwell on the negative influencers in your life since this book is about improving its quality. If I were to focus on negative influences, I think it would not help your journey of ageing.

Trudy looked back on her school days with fond memories. She was a bright pupil with a thirst for learning, and when it was recognised by her teachers, she blossomed.

Mr Conlin was one of those teachers. He taught science, and his appearance somehow mirrored his profession. He had a shock of red hair that seemed to have a life of its own – an unruly mess perched on top of a dome-shaped head. His glasses were perched on the end of his nose, and as he peered out of them, his eyes enlarged and became like two laser-sharp probes you could not ignore.

Despite his appearance, his enthusiasm for his subject showed no bounds. He taught his pupils how to think in a much wider way than the routine science textbooks in front of them. Trudy loved his classes. She would come home and beg her mother to take her to the technical library so that she could further this thirst for knowledge – a flame that had started to burn inside. Yes, Trudy got a first-class degree in engineering and ended up leading a team based on an oil rig in the North Sea.

But it is not always to do with academic excellence. Zena was often over at her grandfather's house as she grew up. He was a keen horticulturist and had a magnificent garden which he tended with much care. Bill, her grandfather, enjoyed Zena's visits because it meant he could spend time in his beloved garden teaching his granddaughter the importance of looking after the plants.

Zena never forgot those precious moments of carefully feeling a leaf or a flower, being taught the different elements of planting a seed, watching how it had grown and learning to understand the pollination with the local bees. She realised that her grandfather was such an inspiration to her, and she would never forget the legacy of respecting plants and flowers.

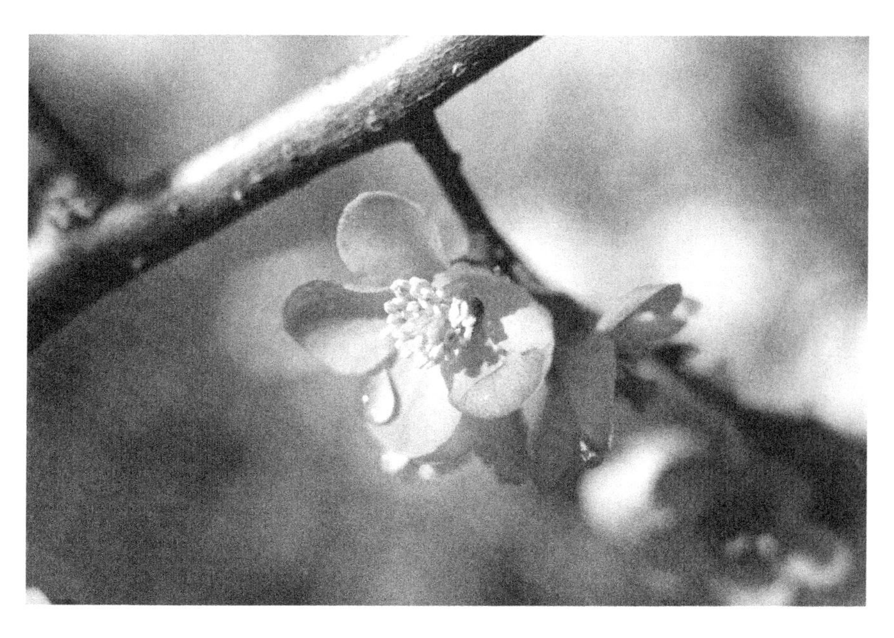

You can gain inspiration from inanimate objects. Mary adored her house. It was a cosy cottage near the coast. When her husband died three years earlier, she decided to move away from the memories of the family home and take up residence close to the Ayrshire coast. What inspired her about the house was that she actually did a lot of the organisation of the construction to make it habitable and designed it exactly the way she thought it should be.

The brochure had said 'needing some work', That was a bit of an understatement. When she arrived, she could see that the roof was full of holes. There was a damp smell from the walls and the garden was a bit of a wilderness. Her first task was to find out about local builders and craftsmen and getting testimonials from neighbours she felt meant she wouldn't be fleeced. Have you ever been in a situation where a company, realising they were dealing with a woman on her own, would sometimes take advantage of the situation?

So, armed with lots of local information (she had got the names of tradesmen from the owner of the local pub), she sat down and planned all the work as to how her cottage would develop over the next few months. Eight months later, yes, she was inspired, the cottage was now the sort of picture you would see in a Homes and Gardens brochure. Of course, the garden needed special consideration since it had been trampled on. It was the dumping ground for building materials and the heavy plant vehicles that were needed when replacing the roof, left it in a sorry state. Inspiration for the garden came from pouring over gardening magazines, listening to gardening programmes on radio and television and even getting inspiration from quirky ideas from the Chelsea flower show.

Many artists talk about being inspired after waking up from a dream - maybe in the middle of the night and rushing to write down what has come into their mind.

I don't know if you have had what you thought was a brilliant idea at night, only to find that you've completely forgotten about it by the morning. If you want to use the amazing power of your thoughts, then have a pen and pad by your bed. When you wake up, write down anything that you remember. Sometimes it may not make sense, but other times it can help you be inspired.

Have you ever attended an evening event and listened to a speaker who inspired you? Maybe it was something that was said, but certainly, there will be an emotional component to the words. It may be a good idea to reflect on that and, in some cases, move in a certain direction. 'If she can do it, so can I.' Inspired women are usually happy, and is not that one of the most important states to be in?

Often a disabled person will talk about their story, the trials and tribulations and the determination to make a difference despite the handicap. Individuals who have lost limbs, hands, feet in war or after sepsis, talk about inspiring moments dealing with adversity.

Instead of going through life blaming whomever or whatever for their situation they often become public speakers. By speaking out, their stories can inspire thousands of people to go out and live their dreams despite major setbacks.

When you're over 50 is it too late to pursue your dreams? I do not think so. Listening to people like Rhonda Byrne author of 'The Secret' and Jack Black a Glaswegian and author of the 'Mindstore' you are guided through imagery to plan your life and imagine the life you want is actually in place.

Many disbelievers talk of gold bars coming out of the sky and hitting you on the head making you rich but writing goals down and then planning the journey in imagery can work.

Imagine waking up every morning feeling inspired with a real purpose in life?

You can do that by engaging your mind in a positive way.

TIPS AND THOUGHTS

1. Become inspired by something or someone.
2. Try out a technique to propel you towards that quality in your life.

chapter 12

F is for Fats

Fats always seem to be in the headlines these days. One minute you are told they are bad for you then an article appears about why you need to include a sufficient quantity in your diet. The following unravels the myths about fats and why I think taking an omega 3 supplement is worthwhile for a woman over 50.

Omega 3 is an essential fatty acid, but I thought I would start off by discussing the different types of fats and why omega 3 is one of the important ones.

Trans fatty acids

Trans fatty acids are produced when vegetable oils are hydrogenated. This chemical process causes the oil to become solid. An example of a product is margarine. The food industry welcomes this type of fat because it lasts longer without 'going off' and, because of its consistency, it works well in baking and even deep-frying.

But your body regards these trans fatty acids as 'foreign'. They actually lower the levels of 'good' cholesterol and, therefore, increase the risk of coronary heart disease.

There are also reports that they can increase inflammation which again may cause heart disease and possibly increase the chances of developing asthma. I suggest cutting these types of fats out of your diet completely.

Omega 6 fats

The western diet is generally overloaded with omega 6 fats. Examples are corn, soy, sunflower and safflower oils. Generally, the ratio of omega 3 to 6 is out of step for ideal health. This should be 1:1 but in many cases, it can be over 1:20. If you take too many omega 6 fats then it can cause ill health. Some examples are heart disease, cancer, depression, Alzheimer's disease to name but a few. Getting your ratio into balance can improve your health.

It has also been reported that heating these oils transforms them into trans fatty acids which, as I have already stated, should not be digested and should be avoided at all costs.

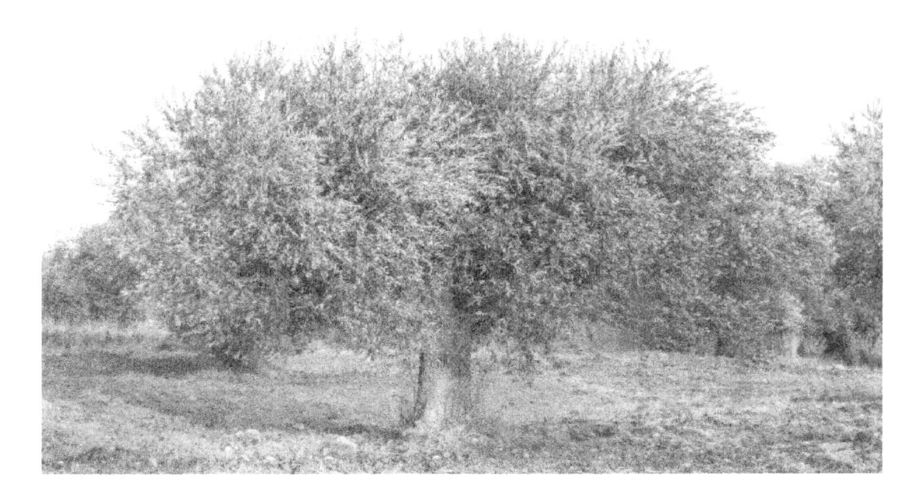

Olive Oil

This is a monosaturated fat and is good for your health because it contains several nutrients including vitamins A and E. It is obtained from the fruit of olive trees. This is an unprocessed oil, meaning it hasn't been heated. To get the best from it, it should be used uncooked e.g.

on salads. It is an omega 9 fatty acid and I suggest to get all the benefits from this oil you should use extra virgin olive oil. It is an unrefined oil that is packed full of antioxidants and anti-inflammatories. (Remember - inflammation in the body can lead to disease). It should be kept away from the light because it can deteriorate quickly if not stored correctly, but that is its only fault - it has many health-giving properties.

Saturated fats

Saturated fats have generally got a bad name in terms of heart disease. If, however, you look at some races around the world whose main diet consists of meat and milk, you find they have low cholesterol levels. Examples of foods that contain saturated fats are meat, dairy and confectionery.

These fats are very stable at high temperatures. They do not become rancid and alter with heat to become trans fatty acids. One saturated fat I particularly like is coconut oil. I buy good quality organic coconut oil for cooking because I know it will not become toxic.

I do not know if you have heard of the 'pulling' effect of coconut oil. Moving coconut oil around your mouth for about 20 minutes then expelling it into a rubbish bag (not the sink where it will solidify and block the pipes) will reduce the build-up of plaque. Plaque causes halitosis, plus untreated, it can be the main cause of gum disease - injurious to health and could result in loss of your teeth.

Omega 3

Omega 3 is an essential fatty acid. The word essential tells us just that - it must be obtained from our food or supplements. The best source of omega 3 is from oily fish.

Examples are:

- Mackerel
- Kippers
- Salmon

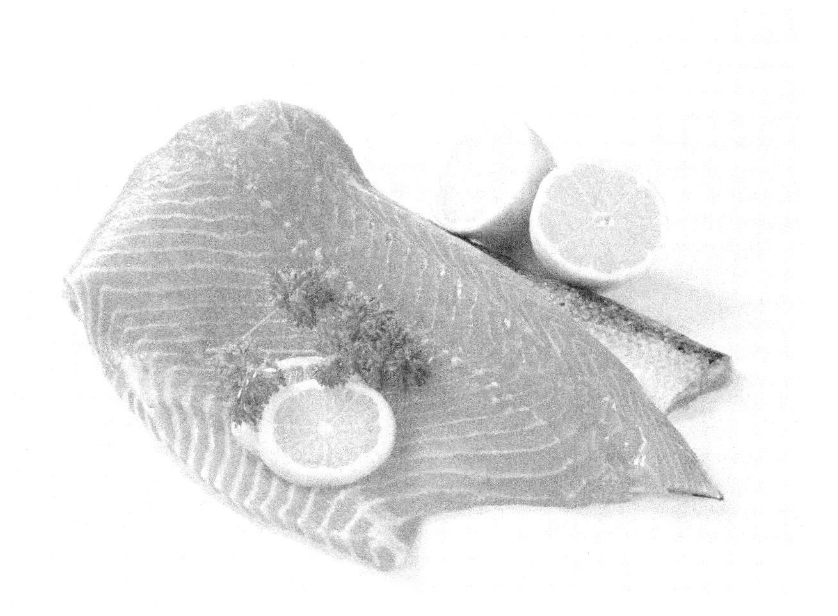

- Fresh crab
- Herring

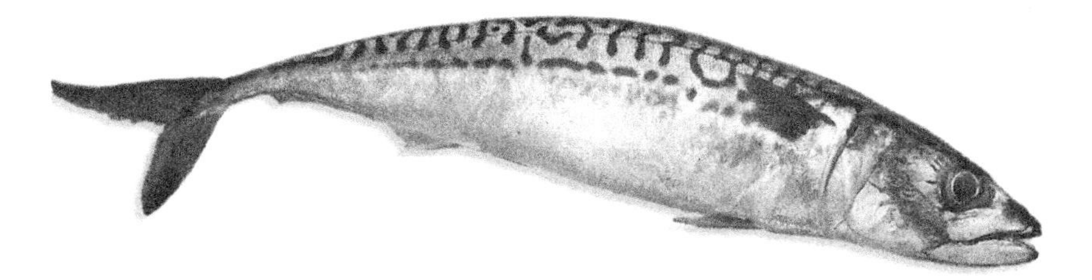

- Sardines
- Whitebait
- Swordfish

- Haddock
- Cod
- Plaice
- Dover sole
- Red mullet
- Shark

Omega 3 consists mainly of two components EPA and DHA. These two components are in your brain tissue, the retina (back of the eye), adrenal glands and sex glands.

Let us look at how this essential oil is beneficial to your heart. If you were unlucky enough to have a heart attack or stroke, then what was happening was that the blood platelets had become sticky. With EPA and DHA, the components in omega 3 reduce the clotting possibility in blood and arteries.

One of the measures of your heart health used by most health professionals is your cholesterol level. Taking omega 3 can lower triglyceride levels and the 'bad' cholesterol component of your blood.

Blood pressure can be lower and because of the effect on certain hormones, the clot-forming property of the oil reduces blood platelets from clumping together.

Skin, nails and hair

In order to have strong nails, glossy hair and silky skin, you need to be taking essential oils. You can rub creams and oils on your face but to get your skin nourished to the point where it feels softer and smoother, your body needs to have an adequate level of essential fatty acids. The same applies if you want to have fewer wrinkles and have a youthful complexion. There is also a body of evidence that suggests that one of the nutritional components required to protect the skin from the damaging effect of sunlight is essential fatty acid-rich oils. I say one of the components because you need to have a diet that includes vitamin E, C, A and minerals such as selenium, zinc and sulphur. Dr Budwig, a researcher, even suggests that it is a deficiency in the essential fatty acid oils that contributes to skin cancers caused by sun exposure.

Arthritis

Arthritis is a pain in the joints and muscles where there is bone deterioration and inflammation. This can cause stiffness and pain. The essential fatty acids are required to lubricate your joints and are also needed to build bone and help move minerals to where they are needed.

Often pain in the joints can lead to giving up sports and, worse case, starting to live a sedentary life. Regular exercise, as well as increasing metabolic rate, which means you burn more calories, also helps you lose the fat which is causing weight gain in most women.

Eyes

Research has shown that omega 3 may have a protective effect on macular degeneration. This condition is a deterioration of the macula in the back of the eye. The first thing you might notice is, when looking at a square object, the sides appear deformed. What is happening is you are starting to lose your central vision so that in acute cases you can only see out of the sides of the eye. The vision becomes more and more blurred until you have difficulty making out faces. As well as omega 3, I suggest you supplement with lutein and zeaxanthin and, of course, your diet should be full of different coloured vegetables. Eggs and spinach seem to have the highest proportion of these two substances.

Menopausal symptoms (See Chapter 7)

You, like many women, may find menopause a difficult time. As well as life changes, for example saying goodbye to the family, leaving the house empty and quiet, there are symptoms in your body that can take over your life. Hope is at hand though.

In 2009 a group of Canadian researchers found that the symptoms of depression and hot flushes were reduced when these women supplemented with omega 3.

Although omega 3 is required for our brains, studies have not shown categorically that it does improve cognitive function. I am taking it anyway.

I have tried to explain that not all fats are bad, in fact, there are benefits as well as essential fats that your body needs for optimal health.

THOUGHTS AND TIPS

1. Look at what you are eating in terms of fats.
2. Are you eating a balance of good fats?

Chapter 13

E is for Exercise

Do you think you need to do exercise?
I thought I would start with what exercise does for your body.

Exercise means you take more oxygen into the lungs. Every cell in your body needs oxygen to produce energy for its work. When the oxygen is taken into your lungs, it is transported in the circulating blood by haemoglobin. It is then delivered to all the cells while their waste product, carbon dioxide, is collected by the blood and transported back to your lungs to be breathed out. The circulation is maintained by the pumping action of the heart, while the movement of muscles 'massages' the vessels of the lymphatic system, enabling them to remove waste material more efficiently.

The bottom line is that any activity or exercise improves not only the circulation but waste removal and energy production in your whole body.

Incidentally, Dr Otto Warburg, twice Nobel Laureate, stated that 'the primary cause of cancer is the replacement of normal oxygen respiration of body cells by anaerobic (oxygen-deficient) cell respiration'. In other words, cancer cells thrive in a medium with little oxygen.

But what type of exercise is right for you? Running a marathon is not appropriate for many people, but it might be something you wish to explore.

Two Americans, Jeannie Rice (71) and Betty McHugh (90), each run marathons as part of their lives. I'm giving those examples not because I am suggesting you go out and run a marathon but because many women will just dismiss such a notion as being impossible. Because you are reading this book, I know you are not one of them.

Marathon running in itself is not something I would particularly advocate. There is an increased strain on knees and ankles that can leave you with injuries. I certainly suggest weight-bearing exercise as a way to minimise bone wasting disease, osteoporosis, but walking or bouncing on a rebounder (a mini-trampoline) will bring many benefits. (See below)

If we look at the different diseases that can manifest as a result of inactivity, it is just so important to address this side of your life and get moving.

Just being overweight (a BMI of 25 plus) can cause a 7% increase in all disease burden, according to the World Health Organisation[4]. Heart disease is one of the increasing risks of ageing. Hypertension (high blood pressure) increases with age and, of course, that is one of the risk factors for heart attack and stroke. The good thing is you can reduce your blood pressure with exercise. If you have a blood pressure monitor, it is an idea to check your blood pressure from time to time. Please do not get fixated on the numbers since these fluctuate during the day. About 40% of people with high blood pressure do not realise they have it. It is only when it becomes much higher that dizziness and maybe headaches alert the person that something is amiss.

If you are 50, then you should have a resting blood pressure of ideally 120/80. These numbers depict the systolic (the higher number) - the contraction of the heart and the diastolic - relaxation of the heart. When it reaches 140/90 then normally medication is introduced. The higher your blood pressure, the higher is your risk of stroke. Every 10mm reduction in blood pressure also reduces the risk of heart failure, coronary heart disease and all risk mortality between 13% and 28%.

As well as age, the other risk factors are the sex of the person. A woman like yourself has less of a risk than men up to the age of 65. It then seems to reverse, and women are at greater risk of having high blood pressure.

If you are black or from an ethnic minority, as well as hereditary influences, then you may have a higher risk.

You can modify your risk by stopping smoking, reducing excessive alcohol intake, reducing salt, getting anxiety under control and, of course, increasing your exercise.

So, what sort of exercise is right for you?

A few years ago, I got myself a rebounder - it is a mini-trampoline. In Albert Carter's book, he talks about a family of trampoline artists who exhibited tremendous strength due to their activities. They took up arm-wrestling and found they were fitter, stronger and had improved balance compared with their rivals. Albert himself had a resting pulse rate of 39 (this is an athlete's pulse rate), yet trampolining was the only exercise he took part in. Gravity, acceleration and deceleration are the three components of trampolining that causes these fitness benefits for the body.

It is also the type of exercise that anyone can do. There have been reports of those in a wheelchair placing their feet on the rebounder while a family member bounces on the trampoline so that the wheelchair-bound individual receives some benefit.

Even a small movement - something called the 'therapeutic rock' - standing with bent knees and gently rocking has shown some pain-relieving properties.

NASA uses this type of exercise when astronauts return from space. Having been in weightless conditions for sometimes weeks, they have the start of muscle and bone wasting. Their scientists carried out the first research into the use of trampolines as effective exercising. They studied the amount of G-force experienced at the forehead while exercising compared with the force at the ankle and on the back. These forces were found to be equal, unlike running on a treadmill where the ankle G-force was always more than twice that of the back and forehead. It did, however, produce beneficial effects for bone and muscle.

Resistance training is a type of exercise that is extremely beneficial. A simple exercise is to sit with a tin of beans in each hand. Moving your lower arm up and down with the weights seems to increase telomere length - that is a measure of how old your body is.

Researchers in America took a group of over 65's who had never exercised before and split them into two. The one half was given stretching exercises, and the other half resistance training with weights. What was surprising was that those who did the resistance training were found, through measurement, to be younger.

Many people talk about yoga.

Yoking was a practice used to connect and harness two animals. They would be "yoked" together (typically at their necks) to then be able to perform tasks (such as ploughing a field). So, essentially, to yoke is to create a union, and this is, typically, how we hear yoga defined today.

There are benefits to yoga:
* reduces stress including headaches;
* boosts energy;
* improves balance and digestion, and
* can relieve symptoms of menopause.

There are yoga positions that you should be able to do – just take it slowly at first:

You are best to warm up by rubbing your muscles vigorously. First your arms then down your legs. Also breathing in unison with the exercise is important.

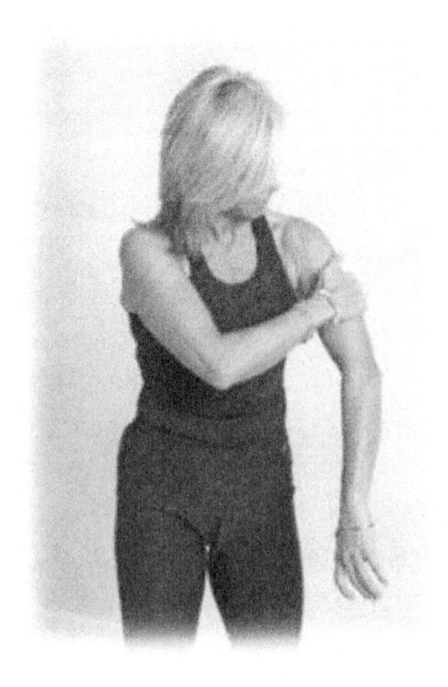

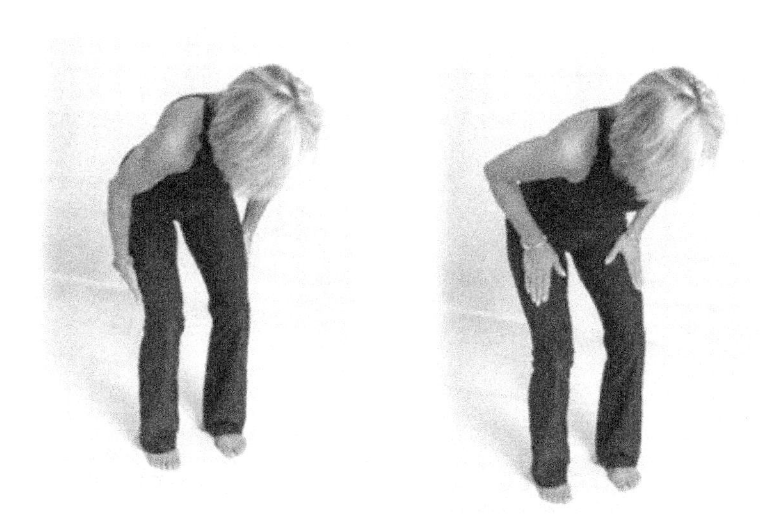

1. Stand upright with your feet together and inhale deeply. Exhale, then press your palms together in front of your chest, touching the skin in front of your heart with the back of your thumbs.

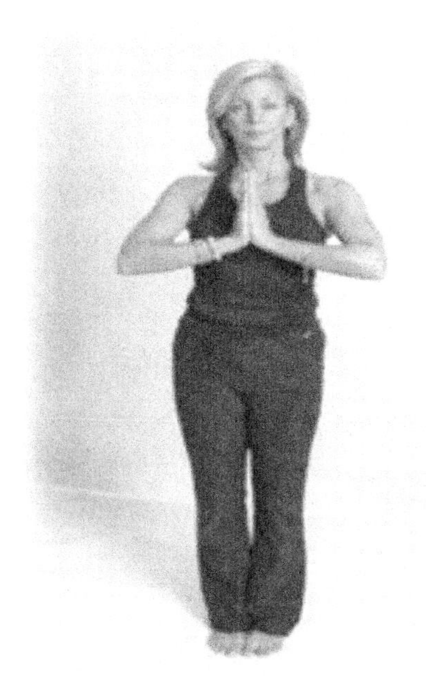

2. Inhale and unlock your thumbs, extending your hands out in front of you. Watch your hands as you raise them above your head and, with knees loose, not locked, lean backwards from your hips as far as is comfortable.

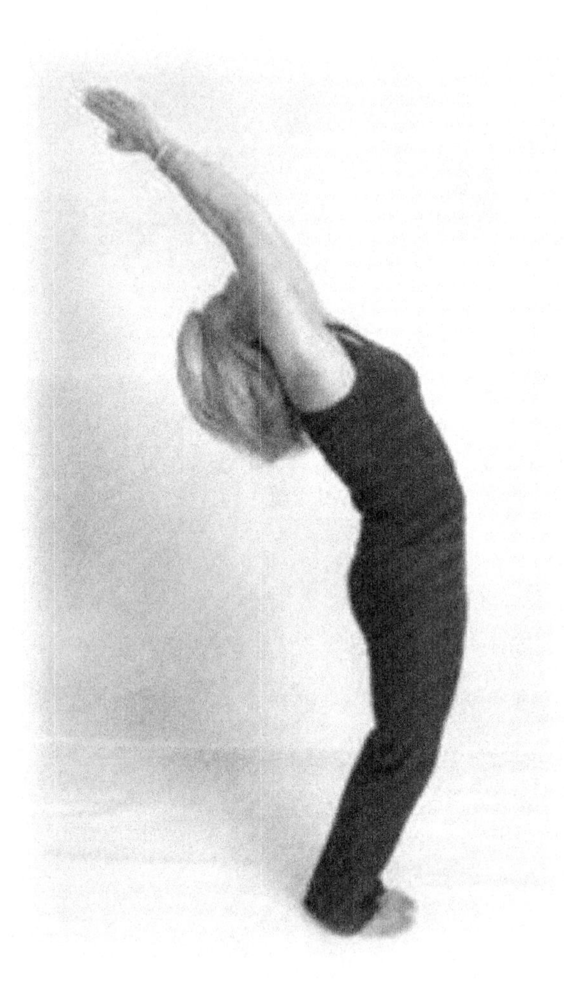

3. Exhale and fold your body slowly forward, from the waist, bending your knees as you go down. Ideally touch the floor with your hands but, if you

are unable to do that, then let your hands hang in a relaxed manner.

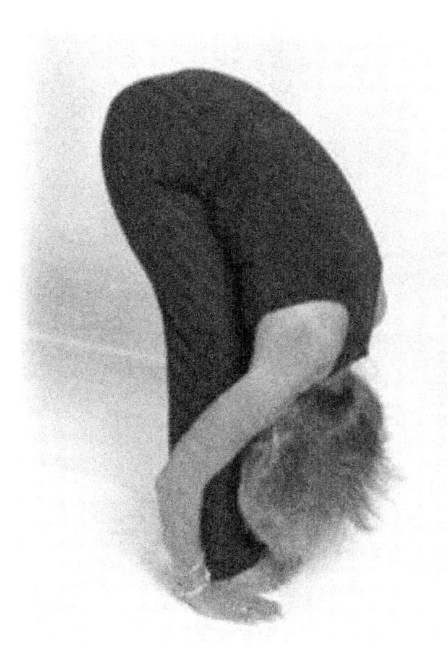

4. Inhale and, bending your knees, place your palms flat on the floor beside your feet. Bring your right knee up, keeping your knee at right angles to your chest and look up. Keep your right foot between your hands and extend your left foot far back and place your left knee on the floor. Bring your right knee up to your chest and look up.

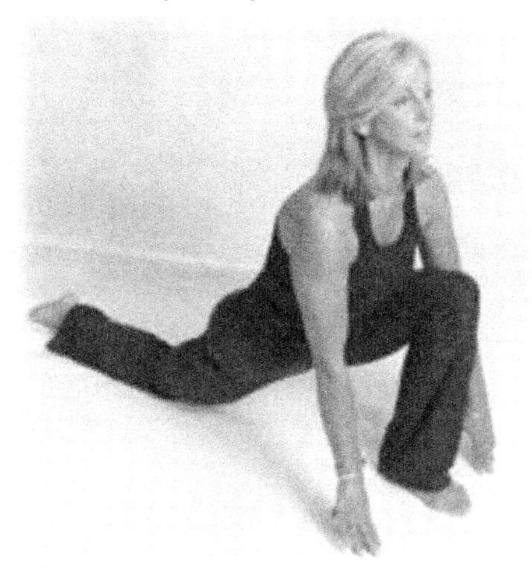

5. Exhale and extend your right foot back to meet your left. Leave your hands where they are. Push your bottom up to make a triangle with the floor. This time look at your feet and lower your heels towards the floor.

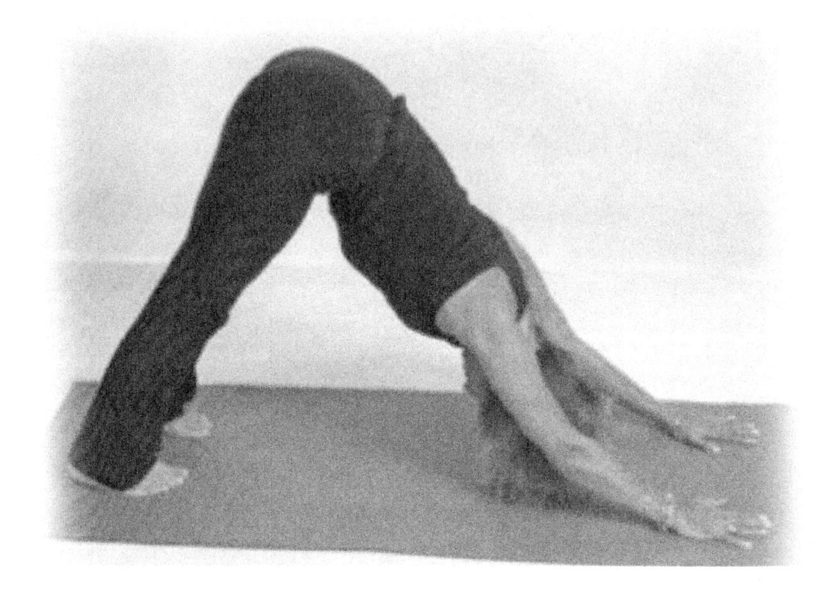

6. When you inhale, lower your knees, chest and chin to the floor, leaving your pelvis raised. Keep your palms beneath your shoulders and your elbows in close to your body.

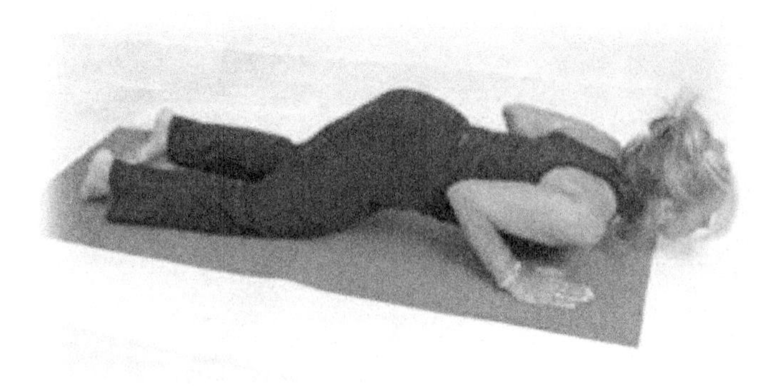

7. Continuing to inhale, lower your pelvis to the floor and let your head and shoulder curl upward like a snake ready to attack.

8. Exhale and push yourself up into the triangle position as in position 5.

9. Inhale again and swing your left foot forward between your hands. Repeat as in step 4 but with the opposite foot.

10. Exhale and swing your right foot forward until it is next to the left foot, between your hands. Straighten your knees while at the same time keeping your arms and hands hanging loosely or flat in the floor.

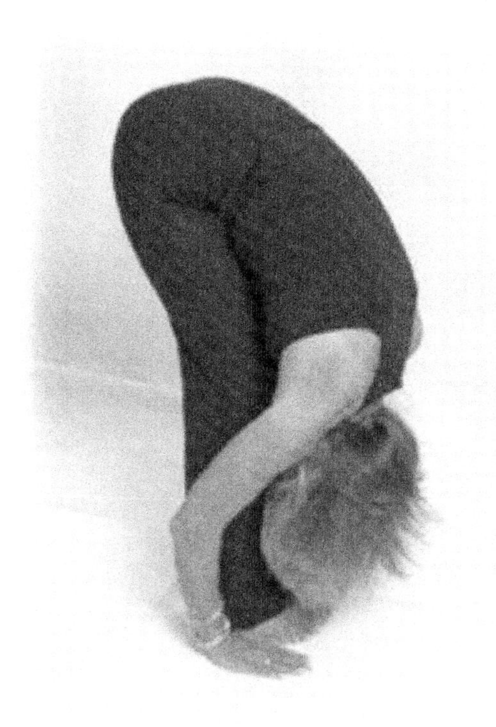

11. Inhale locking your thumbs and unfolding your body slowly until you are in a standing position. Look up at your hands as you keep bending backwards as far as is comfortable.

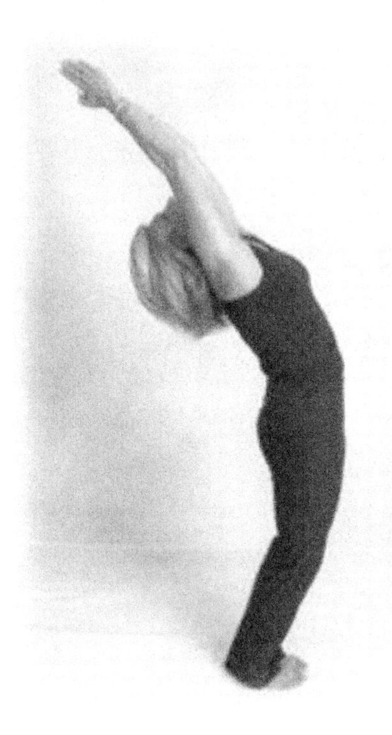

12. Exhale and slowly bring your palms together in front of your chest, the thumbs touching the skin in front to your heart.

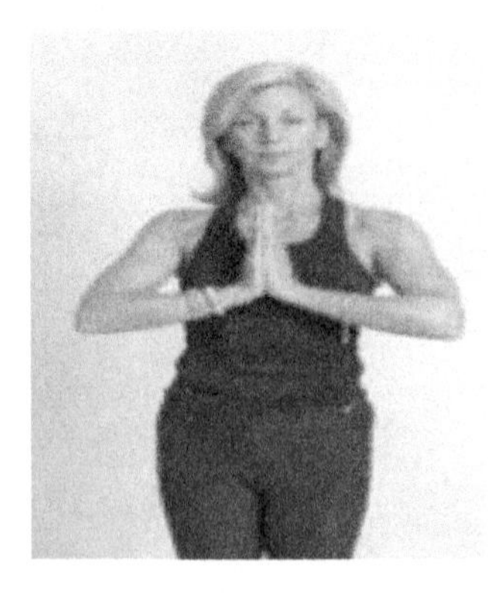

13. Take a deep breath and relax before repeating the exercise. Ideally you should repeat the exercise 7 times. At the end, lie flat on your back with palms at your side facing up and listen for the controlled beat of your heart. Information on classes and training can be found at the back of the book.

Can simple walking be good for you? The answer is yes. NHS (UK) advice is 150 minutes a week, i.e. 30 minutes a day for five days in the week. This can be as simple as going for a brisk walk. Research has shown there is a marked reduction in the incidence of dementia when exercise is introduced as an ongoing routine. Many researchers talk about 5-6 miles a week.

But how can exercise be enjoyable?

Suzie decided enough was enough. She had put on weight and was becoming quite sluggish generally. Her friend Jane and she decided to make a pact. Each would, in turn, come to the other's door at a set time during the week (they were allowed weekends off). There would be no excuse, never mind the weather. 'Get extra layers on or wear your waterproofs', said Suzie when she arrived at her friend's house in the pouring rain on a particularly cold night.

So, Jane quickly donned the appropriate clothing-so important - and they headed out into the cold. It was enjoyable because they were able to chat about everything that was happening in their lives. Each of them had recently taken earlier retirement, so they compared notes on what they were doing with their lives now that they had some time. 'I'm thinking of volunteering for charity work', said Suzie, and they talked about what sort of charity resonated with her and where she would find real fulfilment in the next part of her life. Both of them wrote down in a diary what they had achieved regarding their exercise. For Suzie, it was about getting fitter and watching what she was eating, maybe a reduction in her weight? For Jane, she felt the exercise and the camaraderie was just uplifting and looked forward to the time with her friend. Mentally and physically, they both gained so much from this activity.

Sally did not really want to exercise outside, so she decided that dancing was for her. She joined a Zumba class where she exercised with a group of women once a week. In between, she could be seen dancing in her kitchen to her favourite music.

Having been brought up in the '60s and '70s she knew every word of the Beatles, Mo-town and the Rolling Stones numbers. With the blinds down and the music blaring out, she danced about, oblivious to how she looked, but thoroughly enjoyed the experience.

Have you ever heard of exercising on a vibration plate? You will find these contraptions in some gyms although there are now smaller versions available for a home purchase.

It is a machine designed to stimulate muscles that are being worked by sending high-speed vibrations through the body. When you stand on a plate it feels as if your whole body is being stimulated. Because your muscles are being worked at much higher rates it is claimed that it is a powerful way of toning and strengthening muscles in a short time. It is worth a try if you are game.

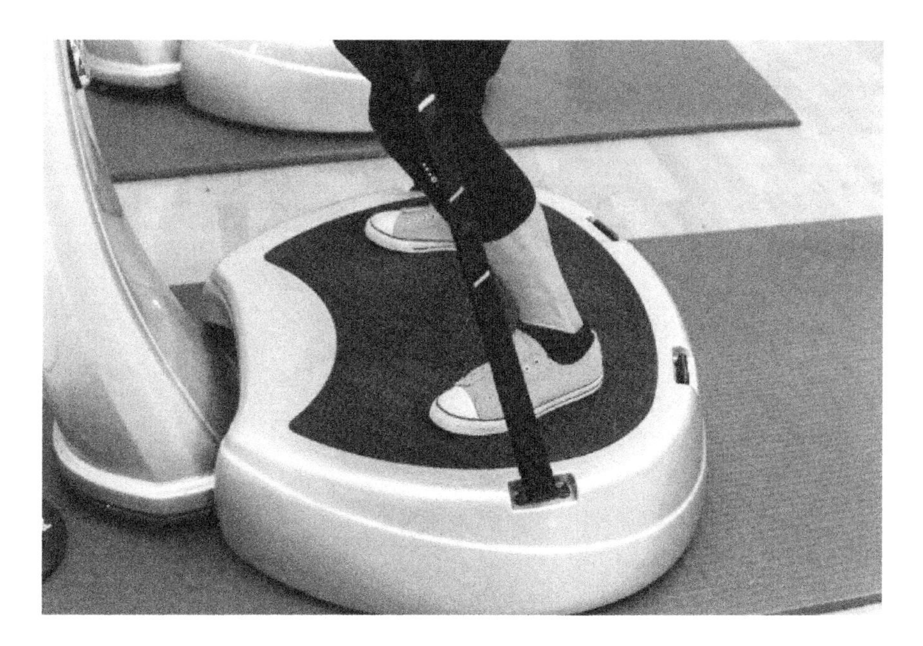

Coldwater swimming seems to be gaining momentum. It is supposed to have health benefits for example a boost to the immune system and a lower incidence of respiratory tract infections, but remember a sudden shock to the system could precipitate a heart attack. On the positive side, a protein released by the body when it is subjected to a cold shock may delay dementia.

And talking about staving off dementia, racket sports seem to be the best exercise activity for the mind, so all you tennis and badminton players, keep it up.

I want to finish with something called Peak 8. Many women say they do not have time for exercise and I am sure that is not you. But in case it is, this type of exercise takes just a maximum of 15 minutes. It is all about getting your heart to a near-maximum rate for a very short time. Running on the spot - maybe on a 'Rebounder', for 60 seconds, then relaxing for 2 minutes and repeating this five times is so beneficial for your body.

We do not often raise our heartbeat in sedentary activities, but this is a way of doing that, and it does not take much time.

In this chapter, I have tried to suggest different types of exercise that are available for you.

TIPS AND THOUGHTS

1. Take some time to decide the correct exercise for you
2. Set aside 20 minutes a day/ 5 days a week for exercise
3. Please enjoy what you do and if you think it's a good idea take a note of what you've done and celebrate.

Chapter 14

S is for Stress

Stress comes in lots of different forms and can be caused by a variety of reasons. Surveys suggest money, work, and health are the main culprits.

Let us, first of all, look at what stress is doing to your body. The fear fight and flight mechanism inherent in everyone was designed to keep you out of danger. In prehistoric times you needed that mechanism to get you out of trouble. When it kicks in there is a flood of adrenaline. Your heart rate increases, your muscles are toned ready to flee, your eyes are wide open, alert and, conversely, your gut takes a back seat and sinks down. To illustrate this - remember a school race - your mouth would be dry, your gut would possibly be champing at the bit and your heartbeat increased ready to propel you forwards. Nowadays, as suggested above, you may experience this sort of reaction when something does not go well at work, you have an unusually high bill to come that comes into the house and you do not know how it happened, or there is a health issue that is just not resolving.

These released stress hormones can be dissipated with exercise, or conversely meditation, but it is probably the last thing you want to do when you are feeling this way.

Stress has a multitude of effects on your body. I talk about increased blood pressure in Chapter 13. You may experience headaches, skin rashes or even overwhelm. Have you ever been in a situation where there has been so much to do that you cannot think straight, your memory goes, and you break down?

There have also been instances of the opposite.

A mother lifted a truck off her daughter using the adrenaline response in her body. Later, going back to the scene, the mother was unable to budge the truck. Yes, the human body can be amazing at times.

The meaning of stress in the Concise Oxford Dictionary is a 'constraining or compelling force' and, therefore, could be constructive or destructive in your life. If you did not have a certain amount of stress, then you might not achieve the remarkable things that you have done and actually are yet to happen in your life.

Chronic stress is definitely something to avoid for health reasons and even premature ageing.

I am a great believer in looking at how you might react or deal with stress. I like the example of someone behind the wheel of a car. At the junction ahead the driver narrowly misses a car that jumped the lights. The rush of adrenaline was intense – he beeped his horn, gesticulated and generally felt a rush of blood to his head. He was angry. Take another person - a woman this time, since I am talking to women. The same thing happens only the woman's reaction is quite different. She accepts that there are crazy drivers about and shrugs her shoulders, no one was hurt, let us get on with the drive. Undoubtedly, the gentleman's blood pressure would rise dramatically and probably stay augmented for some time. The woman on the other hand did not experience the acute response and will ultimately be in better health at the end of the journey.

But, what if it is a person that is causing the stress. Many women in their 50's and beyond are sandwiched in between grown-up children and elderly parents.
Dara was someone that was caring for her mother,

who, although had been extremely independent in her own home was now increasingly deteriorating and, because of a degree of dementia, had taken on an aggressive attitude when dealing with her daughter. Neurolinguistic Programming (NLP) suggests that changing HOW you think can transform WHAT you think. Her mother's change in personality was having a severe effect on Dara. She said she felt like a child and her mother was somehow punishing her. She also thought this was a ridiculous way to feel as a grown woman but could not see a way out of it.

There is a dissociation technique in NLP that changes the person, in this case, Dara, to the observer as if she is in a film observing what is happening rather than being in the film. (The following is another example of NLP).

The first thing Dara had to do was to close her eyes and imagine the sort of interaction she had been experiencing with her mother. She noted how that made her feel. She then imagined a pleasant feeling in her life and became totally associated with that pleasant feeling, stepping inside herself while looking out experiencing the sights and sounds.

This is where the movie comes in. She imagined talking with her mother in this movie inside her head but totally remote from herself. She then associated the pleasant feelings to this movie and continued the pattern several times until it became automatic. The secret was to 'disassociate' herself from the hurtful interaction with her mother. This meant her stress levels tumbled and she was able to cope with the situation in a way that was not detrimental to her health.
The above technique has been very useful for dealing

with funerals. You dissociate from the actual funeral, looking at what is happening as if you are in a film. This has meant certain women can get through the trauma and acute grief in a dignified way.

Have you ever been for a massage? I remember experiencing an amazing one in Fiji. First of all, it was performed by a young man with just a revolving sheet behind a wicker screen on the beach. Some masseurs have an amazing touch and this particular one had been hired by celebrities who came from all over the world to stay in this particular place.
After the massage, I had a shower in the 'buru' as the

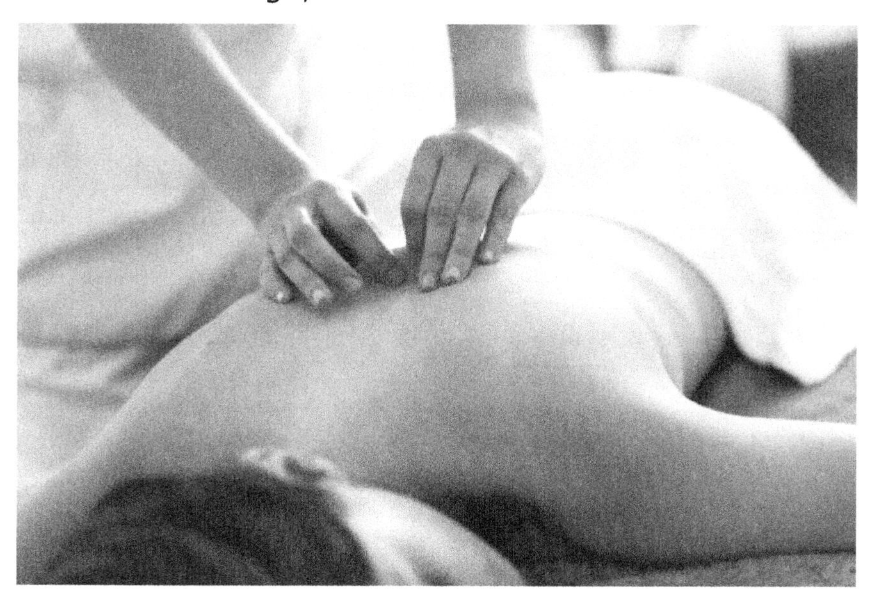

wooden luxury rooms were called. The shower was half in the room and half overhanging the sea. What I remember was that it seemed that each droplet was stimulating nerve endings in my skin meaning my body felt as if it was glowing. An exhilarating experience.
We know that massage can destress the body. It stimulates the lymphatic system producing toxins and that is why you need to drink plenty of water

afterwards to flush the toxins through the body. Just having that half-hour to yourself and experiencing another human being's hands massaging your back can make you feel very relaxed.

TIPS AND THOUGHTS

1. Reducing stress in your life can help you lead a quality life.
2. Dealing with stress in a different way may make you feel happier and also improve your health.
3. Think of ways that are pertinent to your life and start now.

Chapter 15

Y is for being happY

What is happiness? The Oxford dictionary provides the following meaning: 'feeling or showing pleasure or contentment'.

So, what is happening in the body when you feel happy? Researchers from Kyoto University[5] found an area in the brain that was stimulated when participants felt elated. They also found those participants had larger stimulated areas in the brain after being affected by laughter.

The Journal of Neuroscience[6] found that laughter was contagious and formed strong relationships. You have probably experienced that 'having a laugh together' often bonds friends just going through that pleasurable sensation at the same time.

Scientific reports[7] have found there is an increase in oxygen to the brain through a boost in circulation. The immune system is augmented and laughing is similar to a short burst of aerobic exercise. If you laugh and enjoy learning, then there is a transfer of memory from short term to long term.

What does happiness mean to you?

Is it family, friends, or even possessions? You might think that possessions are rather shallow but if you have worked hard to buy something then that can be justified.

I have divided 'to be happy' into its constituent letters.

H is for home. Have you ever felt that feeling of

nostalgia when you have been back to where you grew up? Hopefully it is a good feeling and those memories have shaped your life in a productive way. If for any reason your home does not produce good memories, then there are techniques for altering a memory so that it does not cloud the present. It is a case of describing what you see when you think of it - the modalities. (This is slightly different technique from those mentioned earlier.) Is the picture black and white? Is it moving or static? Are there any noises associated with it? You have then got to change these modalities to the opposite, for example colour for black and white, movement instead of being static and a certain noise unlike the one you remembered. The technique is similar to scratching a record. You are deleting the bad memory and replacing it with a good one.

A is for association. Associating to a happy event in your mind can almost instantly improve your mood. I often use this technique where someone is wanting to change the way they feel.

1. Sit with feet flat on the floor with hands face down on your lap.
2. Take a few deep breaths and then close your eyes.
3. I want you to go back in time, keep going back until you find a moment in your life where you felt total contentment. (For some women it can be holding their baby for the first time and for others it is receiving a well-deserved award etc.).
4. When you are there back in time, I want you to see what is happening, hear the noises of that time and feel, really feel what that was like.
5. When you have truly associated then you press your thumb and finger together and lock that experience in.

6. You then open your eyes and completely disassociate - for example, think about what you're going to eat for lunch.
7. You need to do this exercise three times.
8. To check if you can recreate the feeling press your finger and thumb together and you should experience that scenario again.

P is for parenthood or, if you do not have any children, your own parents. What are you most proud of thinking about how you brought your children up? I am sure that will bring happiness into your consciousness. Watching your children thrive can be a rewarding thought. But, if you see one of them struggling maybe you can use something from the book to help. (If you do not have children then think of how you were brought up).

P is for Personality. One of the definitions of personality is a 'distinctive personal character'. I know that upon meeting someone who seems to have a similar personality to yours you are, more likely than not, to be drawn to that person. The opposite is also true - if you are a quiet individual and meet someone with an abrasive character, forthright and loudly spoken, you will probably be repelled.

Is it possible to change your personality? Research tells us that you may have changed your personality simply in relation to your age, where each age brings dramatic differences to your personality. Actively engaging in behavioral changes can result in substitution of unwanted traits. It has also been found that dramatic events can mean personalities alter, for example, getting married or bereavement.

Those with higher self control seem to have healthier

lives. If you would like to take a personality test, the one with the most credence is The Big Five Inventory-2 (BFI-2). This test looks at the most common five personality traits:

- Extroversion,
- Agreeableness,
- Conscientiousness,
- Negative Emotionality, and
- Open-Mindedness.

If you are happy with your personality then I am pleased for you but if you are not, it is not too late to change, if that means you lead a happier life.

Y is back to yourself. I talk a lot about YOU in these chapters. You can have the life you desire - remember that.

<u>THOUGHTS AND TIPS</u>

1. What makes you happy?
2. Can you do more of that?
3. Try the exercise on creating happiness whenever you wish.

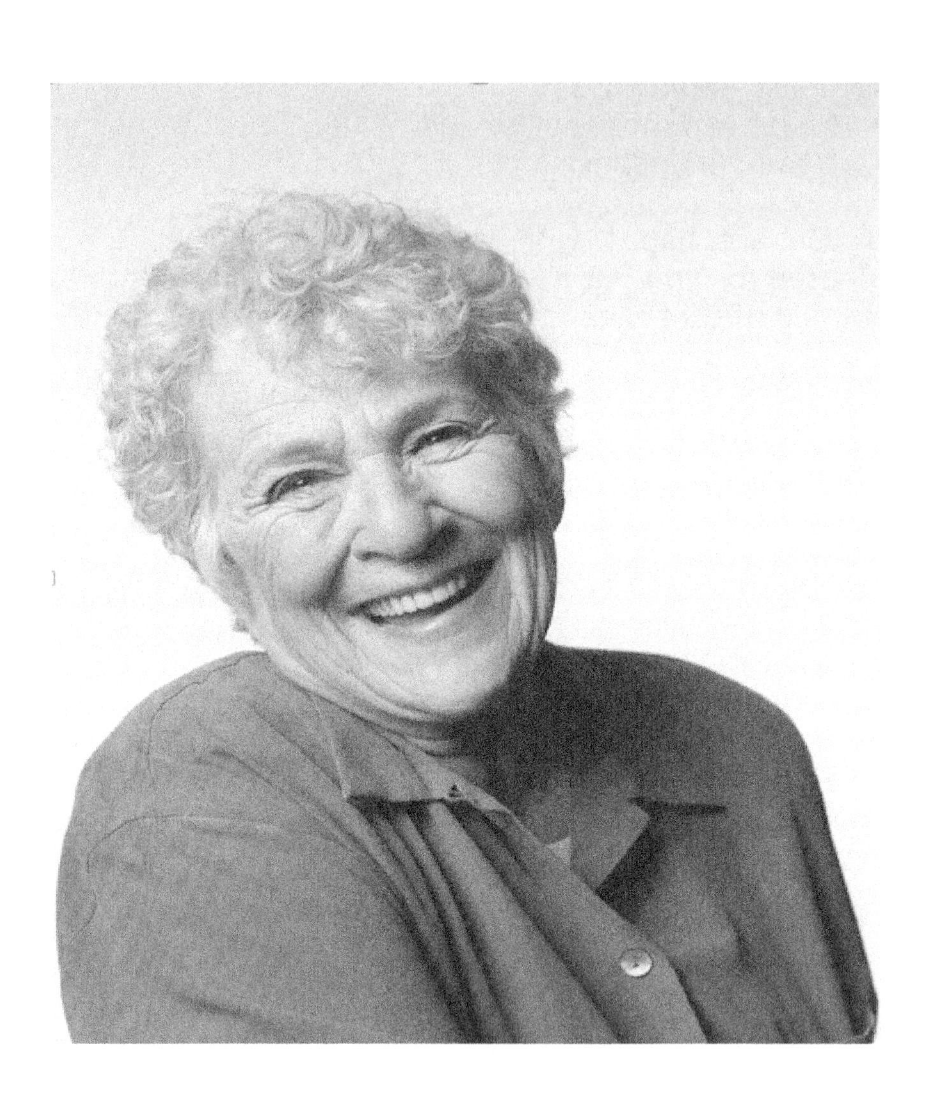

Chapter 16

S is for SUPPLEMENTS

Are supplements really required? There is a lot of adverse publicity regarding supplements but with modern processed foods sometimes coming across continents before eaten, many foods are lacking in the total nutritional value you need for optimal health.

Even looking at soil quality. Many agricultural areas are over-farmed - not allowing the soil to recover and regenerate. Research looking at selenium in soil in the UK found many were deficient.

The use of pesticides and chemicals can sometimes mean the plant is unable to fully utilise nutrients in the soil.

Antioxidants are used in the body to fight free radicals. Cellular decay and tissue damage are thought to be caused by free radicals and that in turn causes ageing. An example of free radical damage in fruit is when you cut an apple in half, it turns brown or steel that rusts. So, antioxidants appear to repair that damage and as I suggest, you probably do not get sufficient quantities in our food. Naturally, antioxidants in the body decrease as you age.

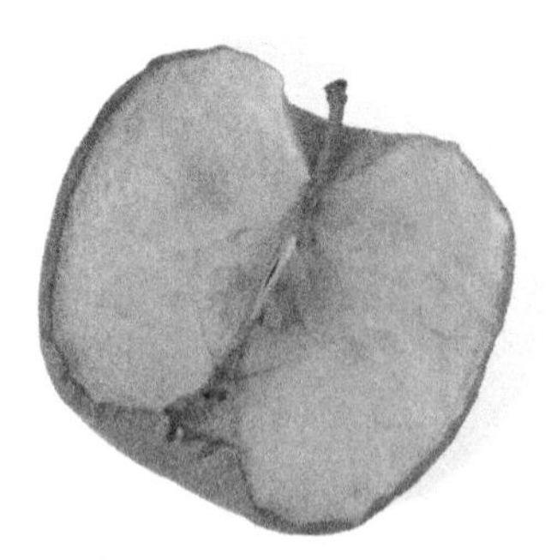

Vitamin C is one of the most common antioxidants but, as explained in an earlier chapter, the amount in foods reduces over time. It is also destroyed by heating, so rhubarb and raspberry tarts may seem to be full of goodness but may contain very little of the vitamin.

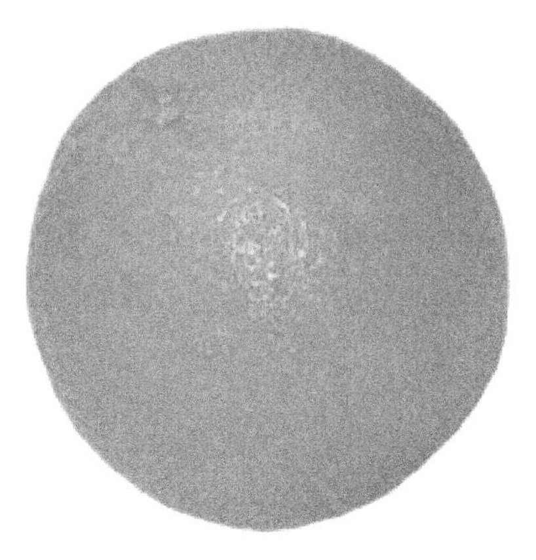

Vitamin B is an important vitamin for the brain. This vitamin can be found in meat and fish but if you are vegan then you must supplement particularly with vitamin B12. Studies from Oxford University gave high doses of three of the vitamin B family B1, B6 and B12 to elderly patients and studied the quantity of amyloid protein present in the brain. It was a double-blind trial so half of the participants were given placebos. Through MRI scans they were able to assess how much of the protein had been accumulated. In the vitamin B cohort, there was a marked reduction in the protein and the significance of this was that, when the brains of Alzheimer's patients were examined, they had an abundance of the protein present. What the researchers did not know was whether giving vitamin B supplements would prevent Alzheimer's. But I think making sure for yourself whether your body has adequate supplies, by diet or supplements, is important. Taking the correct dose is important - check with your healthcare professional.

Do be careful of taking vitamin B6 with some Parkinson's drugs - ask about that if relevant.

Vitamin D is one of the supplements I definitely suggest you take.

Modern lives mean often excessive sunbathing in short bursts. Skin cancer occurs when cells divide too quickly and melanoma or non-melanoma skin cancer such as basal cell carcinoma (BCC) and squamous cell carcinoma can happen. The most common areas for BCC to occur is the face, nose, ears and back of the hands.

Again, the most exposed areas of the skin to the sun can produce squamous cell carcinoma. In prolonged exposure to the sun, damaged cells may not be recognised by the body's defence system and therefore allow them to grow out of control.

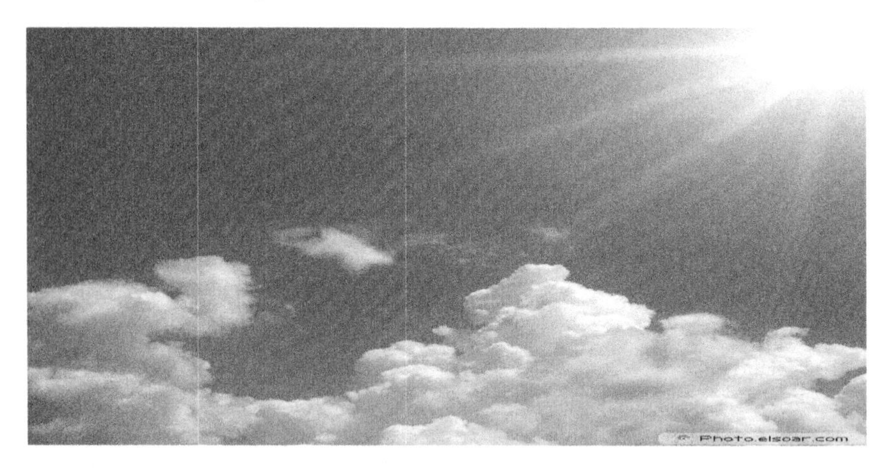

Sensible sunbathing - 15 minutes - until your skin becomes pink is the best way of getting your vitamin D. There are problems, of course, as noted above but also the sun has to be high enough in the sky in order to produce vitamin D on the skin. Northern hemispheres have only a few months of sunshine and, as the angle of the sun is important, it is 11 am until 3 pm that are when we get the most benefit (- the times when we are told to stay out of the sun). You know that you are making vitamin D when your shadow is shorter than yourself. Also, because of cold winds many times you may be outside but completely covered to keep warm.

There are benefits in taking vitamin D for cancer prevention. Breast cancer rates tend to be higher in areas with low levels of winter sunlight. Those women who are exposed to UVB rays (the sun's rays that produce vitamin D in the skin) and consume above average amounts of vitamin D from the diet have significantly lower breast cancer rates. Disturbingly, women who have the lowest vitamin D levels (in the lowest 25%) have a risk of cancer 5 times higher than those with the highest levels.

These are indeed worrying statistics.

Belgian researchers looked at survival rates and size of breast tumours in women and they found that the women with higher vitamin D levels not only had smaller tumours but also had better outcomes - they lived longer. My colleague Dr Helga Rhein, a retired GP who worked in a deprived area in Scotland, routinely prescribed vitamin D for her patients particularly if they had a history of breast cancer. Her findings in terms of reduction in morbidity and mortality rates bore out this fact.

Autoimmune diseases are another area where vitamin D has a role. An autoimmune disease is where the body turns in on itself and breaks down its own tissue. Lupus is an example where virtually everyone with this disease will be low in vitamin D and, unfortunately, going out in the sun can produce skin rashes and a possible relapse of the disease.

Multiple sclerosis (MS) is an autoimmune disease that has links with vitamin D deficiency. In MS the fatty myelin sheaths around the nerves of the brain and the spinal cord are damaged and that means the messages that travel along the nerves slow down. It generally affects young people, especially women. If you have links with MS in your family I strongly urge you to get everyone to take a vitamin D supplement. Allergic diseases such as asthma, rhinitis and eczema are linked to regulatory T cells. The researchers suggest that using either low dose steroids or vitamin D could be used to stop the immune response in these diseases and, therefore, reduce symptoms.

Bone disease is well documented regarding vitamin D deficiency and one of the first diseases linked to that deficiency was rickets. This is a bone softening disease in children and although the diet is a factor in having adequate levels of vitamin D, the main way the body obtains its vitamin D is through exposure to sunlight, specifically UVB rays between 270 and 300mm wavelengths. Osteomalacia is an adult bone disease also caused by vitamin D deficiency. This disease shows itself as muscle weakness with fragile bones causing severe pain.

If you are not getting exposed to sunlight and have reached or gone past your menopause then you are more at risk of broken bones if you are vitamin D deficient.

Other benefits are in coughs colds and chest infections - even Covid 19. The misery of having coughs, colds and flu in winter is not inevitable. We now also know that having higher vitamin D levels can help the immune system when exposed to these new viruses. The number of respiratory infections is generally reduced when vitamin D levels are raised and even if you are unlucky enough to catch a winter bug then it is far less severe when your immune system is up to scratch.

What about doses of vitamin D?

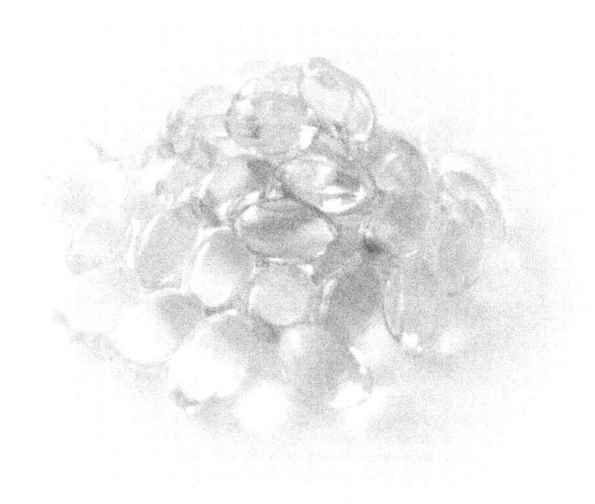

When you go to buy vitamin D the first thing is to make sure you buy D3 and not D2. This is because the D3 type is metabolised differently in the body and will get your levels up quicker.

People ask me about doses. I tend to like to test before suggesting higher doses but if you are a woman in one of the northern countries with little exposure to natural sunlight then I suggest a minimum of 2000iu of cholecalciferol (D3) daily.

What I look to do is to get your levels up to about 100 (25(OH)D) and if you have had cancer, over 100. When we look at the levels of fit young men - lifeguards in Australia, then their levels are around 150nm/l so no, I'm not worried about these higher levels. Of course, you could overdose if you took mega doses and a couple of people with certain conditions should not take supplements: people with hyperparathyroidism, sarcoidosis and those with severe kidney stones should avoid vitamin D supplementation.

What if you are already taking medication?

Generally, it is not a problem. Certain medication for epilepsy, and some diuretics (water tablets), may interact but for specific advice check with your healthcare professional.

Iron is not generally needed and if someone asks me about iron supplementation, usually because they are tired, I suggest getting a blood test. This will tell you accurately what your levels are. Ferrous fumarate 210mg three times a day is normally the initial dose for low iron counts and then usually your blood is checked after 6 months. Often the dose is then reduced and finally stopped.

Iron-rich foods are dark green vegetables and meat.

But, what about the more sophisticated substances - OPC's for example. These are oligomeric proanthocyanidins, one of the most powerful antioxidants. They are present in maritime pine bark and a French scientist, Dr Jacques Masquelier, found they had restorative properties when given to those with nutritional deficiencies. They can be found in fruit such as blueberries.

Grape seed extract and curcumin (turmeric) have also been found to have antioxidant properties. Turmeric is often found in curries, giving it a distinctive yellow colour. Turmeric supplements have been found to be beneficial in dealing with the pain of arthritis.

Vitamin E is found in green vegetables, wholegrain cereals and nuts and works by protecting cell membranes against free radical damage.

If you are thinking of supplementing then I would suggest vitamin D and omega 3 are the two you take. Obviously, I am assuming you are getting the rest of your nutrition from vegetables, fruit and salads particularly in their raw state.

I believe you should get your calcium from your food rather than supplementing it. Vegetables, nuts and fish should give you adequate supplies. You do not need to have dairy to make up the recommended daily amounts.

Probiotics are another emerging supplement. They help to restore the balance of bacteria in the gut. I suggest taking a probiotic whilst you are on an antibiotic since the medication tends to wipe out all the bacteria, not just the ones the antibiotic is designed to eradicate. Supplementing has been shown to reduce diarrhoea with antibiotics and also help with IBS (irritable bowel syndrome). Probiotics are present in food such as yoghurt and non-dairy foods such as sauerkraut, pickles, miso and sourdough.

THOUGHTS AND TIPS

1. Eat a good nutritious diet including raw food.
2. Supplement with vitamin D and omega 3.

Chapter 17

T is for TOXINS

The word toxin, in relation to the body, basically means poison or a disruptive element from the environment which causes cellular damage.

There are certain toxins that we have control over and those that the government has a responsibility to manage. The Clean Air Act of 1956 was brought in to reduce smogs from burning coal, predominantly in household fires. It was to reduce respiratory damage to the lungs, particularly of children living through the 1950s.

In 2020 a coroner ruled that Ella Kissi-Debrah, a 9-year-old who had severe asthma, died as a result of excessive traffic emissions. As I say, governments need to control overall toxins in the environment, but you can also reduce the toxins in your everyday life.

Dr Samuel Epstein, the author of several publications, including 'The Safe Shopper's Bible' and 'Unreasonable Risk', suggests you can reduce your personal toxin overload by taking some action. Before I go into these, let us examine the question 'why is it important to do this?' It is thought that certain products have carcinogenic (cancer-producing) properties.

Dr Epstein lists products that have been proved to be damaging to the skin. Although it has been known for some time that Sodium Lauryl Sulfate, for example, can damage the skin, it can be found in many skin and body products. Aqueous cream used to be a nation-favourite moisturiser but, I suggest that you only use this product to wash dry skin and then remove it. Do not leave it on the skin.

I have talked about free radicals in Chapter 5 but, it seems that toxins in many personal care products and industrial cleaning chemicals may be absorbed through the skin and ingested through the mouth. This has a detrimental effect on health.

Detoxifying your life where possible is definitely something to consider. Choosing to use non-toxic personal and household products could be a start.

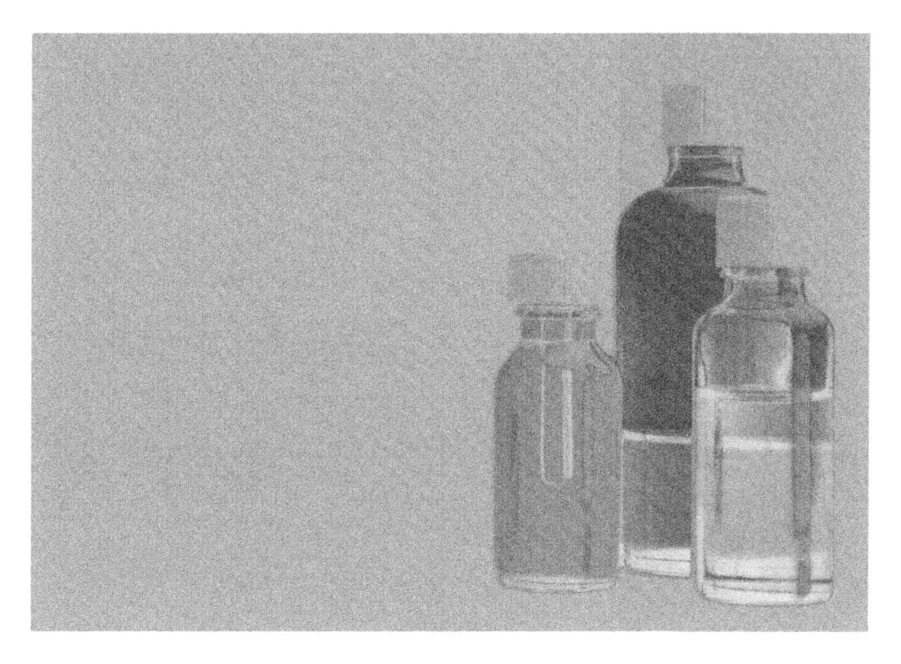

Organic food without pesticides is something to think about. Also, giving your body plenty of fresh vegetables and fruit will increase the transit time in your bowel. Chemical additives, artificial flavouring, and colouring is giving your body more work to do, and the elimination of toxins are essential to keeping your body in great condition.

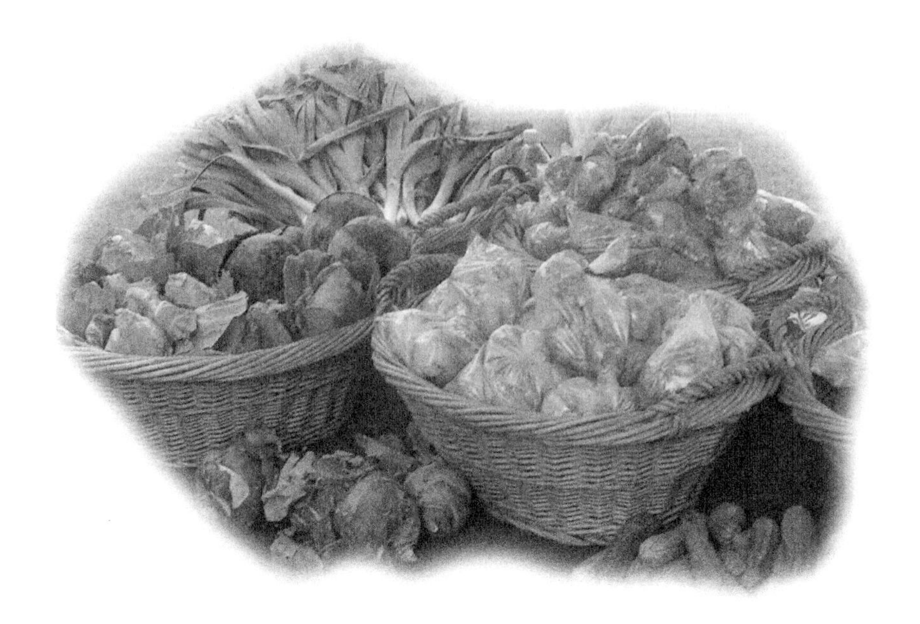

Stimulating the lymphatic system, that is the system that brings nourishment to tissues and takes away waste, is worthwhile. In order to do that, you need to exercise - a brisk walk, a swim or dry skin brushing. Have you ever tried dry skin brushing?

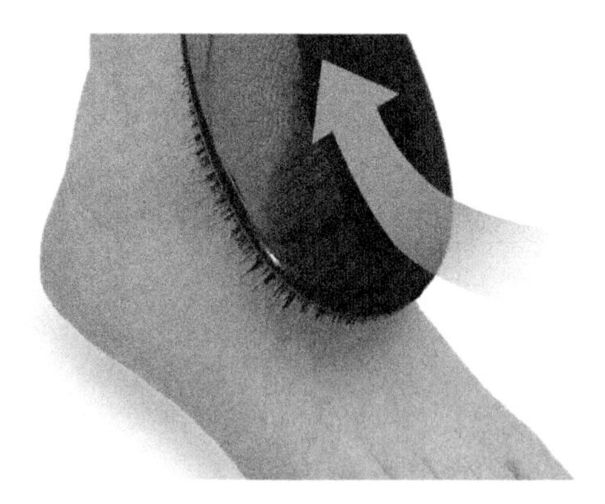

Best to get yourself a good natural bristle brush and start on your feet, brushing upwards, towards your heart. You then follow on, up the legs to the buttocks, then the hands, arms and down the neck and trunk. The neck and upper back should be brushed across the top. I suggest you use this technique three times a week. Experts in lymphatic drainage techniques can massage your body in a way that stimulates lymph dispersal.

There are, obviously, detox diets. They have to be carefully introduced since it can be almost an assault on a body that is full of toxins. Alkalising the body with vegetable juicing can cause unpleasant side effects such as nausea or even sickness. Please don't attempt an extreme diet without professional input.

Another way of detoxifying is colonic irrigation. It is thought that the bowel contains 10-15lb of faecal material (not a pleasant subject) at any one time and ideally, elimination after each meal will make sure transit time is reduced. But with our western diets, our bowels don't generally tell us to defecate sometimes for several days. Colonic irrigation involves inserting a tube in the back passage and pumping warm water into the space to 'clean out' the bowel. Generally, doctors do not advise this procedure but in some cases, with a better diet, it can make you feel energetic.

Last, but not least, Electrical Magnetic Fields (EMF's). They emit radiation that could be harmful to your body. You are surrounded by EMF's and some of the most powerful ionising radiation is from the sun. Certainly, X-rays and MRI scans should be reduced to a minimum. For example, thinking about how you handle your phone that has weak ionisation radiation is important. I mentioned keeping electronic equipment out of the bedroom - is that possible with your phone? Try and keep exposure regarding proximity to your ear, and side of the face, to a minimum and do not keep your phone in a pocket on your person.

THOUGHTS AND TIPS

1. Look at the personal care and household products you are using and replace with non-toxic items.
2. Use dry skin brushing and increase your aerobic exercise.
3. Handle your mobile phone in as safe a way as possible.

Chapter 18

E is for EFT

What does EFT stand for? There are two definitions I have heard of – Emotional Freedom Technique and Emotional Freedom Tapping. I have also heard the term Emotional Thoughtfield Therapy. It is tied to the Chinese body meridians that are also used in acupuncture. It is thought, that by removing emotional ties, healing can take place physically and by tackling limiting beliefs you can achieve peace and fulfilment in your life. Is that something you want to hear about?

So, what research is there available to support this exercise?

David Feinstein[8] has brought together evidence to support the theory. He cites 18 randomised controlled trials that show positive results that are not answered by chance. He states '...the brain gets stuck in an ON position so that the person is continually experiencing the chemistry of being in mortal danger. EFT Tapping turns it OFF!'

The proof, of course, is if it works for you. I do not know whether you think that your beliefs have somehow shaped your life? Those whose self-esteem and beliefs have stopped them from leading the quality life they should be experiencing – 'I am not good enough', 'I do not deserve this' would have been held back.

What if you were able to release this block and start afresh? What if you were to manage pain or emotional blocks and feel free again?

I would suggest you can do that and, if you take time to practice these techniques, you will begin to experience that freedom.

Tara was someone who hated her body. She felt as if she was constantly at war with her weight and her emotions. She started with the affirmation of forgiveness. Forgiving herself and loving herself for who she was had to be at the centre of her healing. This was a very difficult thing for her to do but as she carried on with the affirmations using the EFT technique, gradually she realised that she was sabotaging herself. She said and I quote 'it felt like chains were being lifted from my body, I feel lighter and brighter.'

If any of you are scientists reading this, you may scoff at the idea of emotion being so tied up with afflictions. Is it possible that there is a great deal of emotion within a physical pain? Can a healing of emotions mixed with modern surgery and medicine bring about a greater recovery?

Let us do the technique:

Below are the tapping or rubbing points that need to be addressed in sequence, in order to start the healing process. There is also an affirmation that you might, or might not, want to say:

'Even though I have this belief (whatever it is) I deeply love, forgive and completely accept myself'

And this is said as you tap or rub each of the points in turn.

There is one practitioner, Dr Lee Pulos, who suggests you need to use what he calls a 'circuit breaker' at the beginning of the routine, and also if you are not finding benefit as you go through the process. His 'circuit breaker' is putting three fingers of your left hand on your tummy button and your thumb and index finger of your right hand just under your collar bone and rubbing a few times, focusing on the limiting belief.

You need to decide where it is at the beginning on a scale of 1-10. One being it doesn't bother you, and 10 being it takes up all your thinking. Take a deep breath in and out before you start.

After the circuit breaker, you go round all the points from 1-10 tapping or rubbing, whichever is better for you, saying the affirmation, and checking in halfway through how you feel about that belief now.

DIAGRAM

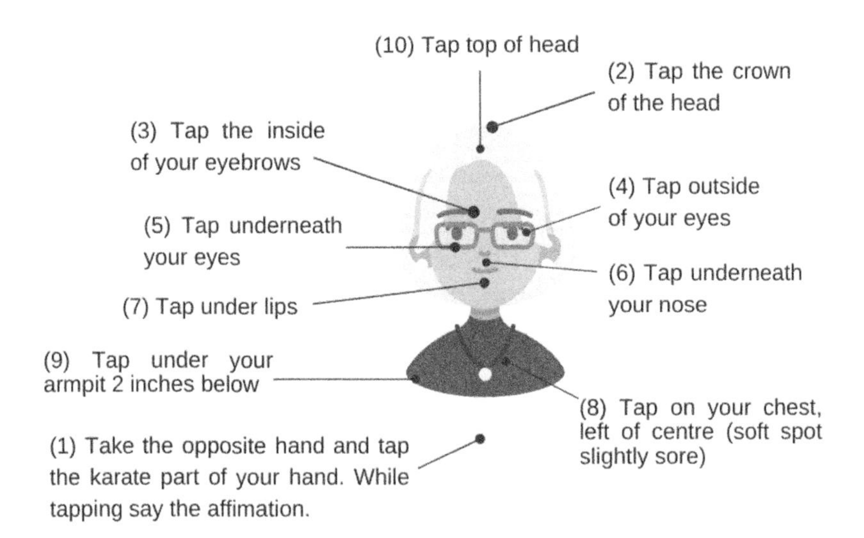

THOUGHTS AND TIPS

1. It is worth trying the technique for unresolved issues.
2. EFT can be a powerful addition to the alternatives available for improving the quality of your life.

Chapter 19

M is for MEDICATIONS

Medication brings up many thoughts with the general population. Should I take medication? Is this medication right for me?

I think it is important to differentiate between the therapeutic side (its efficacy and healing benefit) against the side effects. Prescribers are always striking a balance between these two points.

It is obvious with some disease states that without medication you may well die. I am talking about medication for high blood pressure, heart failure or after a heart attack, to give you just three examples. These disease states unchecked are extremely serious.

There is strong evidence emerging that type 2 diabetes in the main can be eradicated with strict dieting. Many people, however, are on numerous medicines to lower blood glucose, as well as those to reduce blood pressure and cholesterol levels.

Other diseases such as cancer throw up many questions. Will the treatment I am getting cure me? Often it is to put cancer into remission. This is where you can help your body greatly with lifestyle changes and supplements.

Chris Woollams in his book 'Everything You Need to Know to Help You Beat Cancer' shows you how mainstream medicine can work in harmony with alternatives. He does come down pretty hard on sugar, for example.

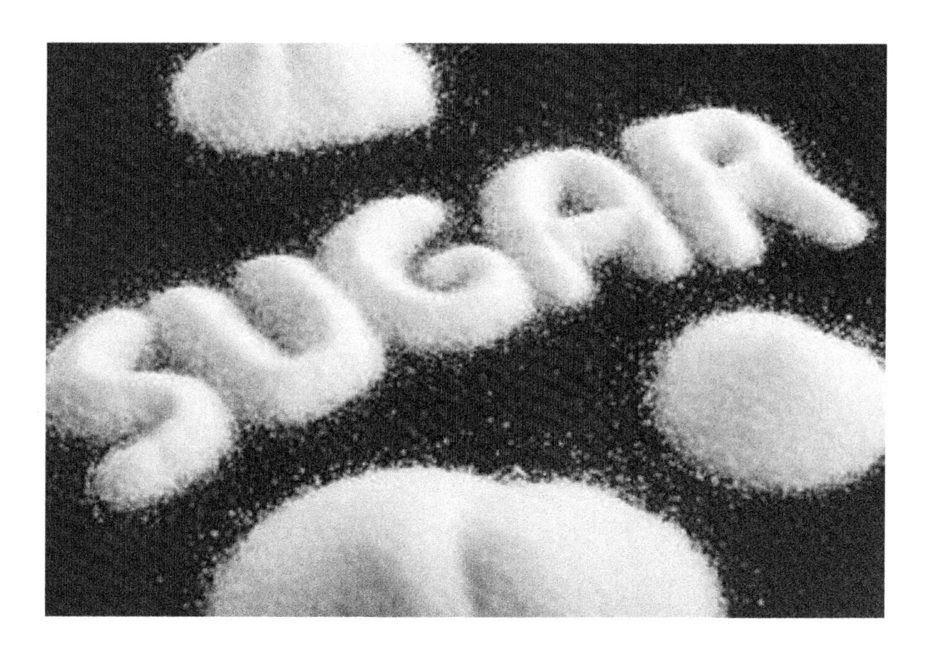

He suggests it needs to be cut out completely. On the other hand, he has shown positive results with supplements in tandem with chemotherapy or radiation.

Taking medicine correctly requires a great deal of detail, hopefully, supplied by your pharmacist. If non-steroidals (e.g., ibuprofen) are taken on an empty stomach, they can cause stomach irritation and, in severe cases, an ulcer. They are, of course, very useful as anti-inflammatories since they reduce pain and stiffness.

Penicillins are sometimes needed to treat an infection. Nowadays, with antimicrobial stewardship, prescribers are urged to prescribe with caution and only when there is a real clinical need. Viruses, for example, are not cured by antibiotics.

What you must do with many penicillins, such as penicillin V or flucloxacillin, is take them when your stomach is empty. Either one hour before food or two hours afterwards. I usually suggest one hour before each meal and one at bedtime. Other antibiotics such as 4 quinolones should not be taken with milk (2 hours apart). Antibiotics are so precious now that to avoid tolerance (where they might not work), they have to be taken correctly.

In the section on osteoporosis, I talked about a weekly medication, a bisphosphonate. That has to be taken either standing up or sitting up straight with lots of water. This is because, if you bend or lie down after taking it, it can cause oesophageal (the tube running from your throat to your stomach) inflammation. It also must be taken well away from other medication.

Shingles can be quite a demanding disease. There is usually a trigger since the virus lies dormant in the body and it appears as a red sore rash on the skin. Often it is when you are run down. The key for the prescriber is to start the antiviral medication, usually aciclovir, as soon as even a hint of a sore rash appears.

This particular medicine has to be taken five times a day and it's useful to give a written timing: 7 am, 11 am, 3 pm, 7 pm and 11 pm. What the medicine does is, hopefully, prevents herpetic (nerve) pain in the future. If the medication can be started right away then that improves the outcome.

But what about taking medication together? There are a few dos and don'ts. An example is iron. Taking an indigestion tablet at the same time can result in the iron not being absorbed properly. Thus the prescriber, when he or she takes the next blood test, may alter the dose upwards not realising there is a problem with the timing of the dose.

Statins, the medicines to take for lowering cholesterol, can increase in concentration in the blood with possible muscle pain, when taken with certain medicines, for example an antibiotic called clarithromycin.

But why do some people not take their medication? There have been studies looking at transplant patients, where it was essential to take the drugs to avoid the transplanted organ being rejected, yet people didn't take them.

An asthmatic who does not take her steroid inhaler regularly can have an exacerbation and end up in the hospital, or worse, lose her life.

When someone dies, often the family bring in carrier bags of unused medicine and you wonder how this has happened. With pharmacists in Scotland now receiving some yearly prescriptions dispensed every 8 weeks for patients, there are many more checks on whether the patient needs a certain medication. With critical medicine, where the prescriber says they need it, the pharmacist will question compliance. Sometimes someone will not take a particular medicine, for example a chewable calcium and vitamin D tablet because they do not like the taste. That can easily be remedied by changing to something that is more palatable.

The returned medicines that are sent back to Health Boards in Scotland reach many tons every year. Imagine if the cost of these drugs could be recouped and put into thousands of hip replacements or to pay for much needed individual costly drugs?

There are many side effects of medicines. Most pharmaceutical companies list side effects according to very common, common, rare, very rare and unknown. Patient leaflets will often cite the side effects. Of course, asking your pharmacist about a side effect that has started soon after a new medicine is added, could result in an explanation being given.

Of course, there are some medicines that have shown side effects some weeks or even months after first use. An ace inhibitor medicine (these are used for high blood pressure) have been shown to cause an irritating persistent cough. A change of medication usually sorts out the problem.

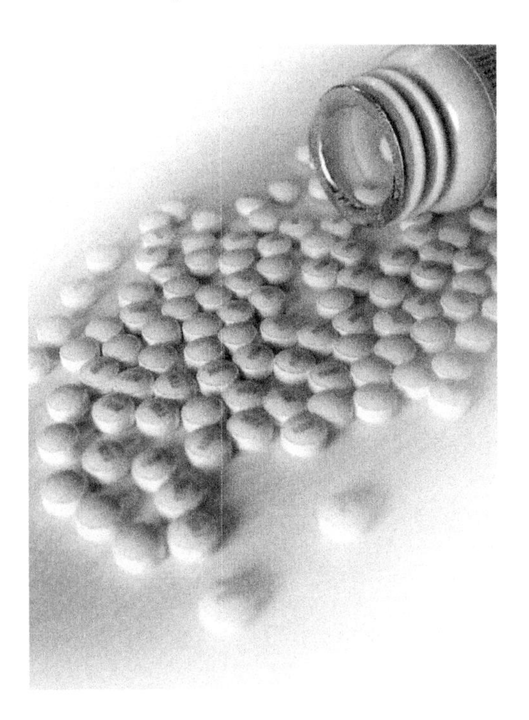

What about certain foods and medicine? Statins (cholesterol-lowering drugs) can become stronger in the blood with grapefruit. Warfarin (for thinning the blood) can again become stronger with several foods e.g vegetables that contain potassium - broccoli or brussels sprouts. Of course, there are many medicines that should not be taken with this medicine and your pharmacist will help with that.

THOUGHTS AND TIPS

1. Make use of your pharmacist to help you understand your medicine and reduce side effects.
2. The future of medicines will be targeted, individualised drugs.

Conclusion

Conclusion

This book is all about improving the quality of your life. Maybe you have learned something new, possibly a technique to try out?

Because women over 50 are diverse, not everything that is written here will resonate with you, but I know you will find some answers for the way ahead.

I am certainly happy to work with you one-to-one to develop the life you want and heal some of the rough patches developed over the years.

You can contact me through the ER Quality Life website, at www.erqualitylifesystem.com.

For information on vestibular exercises go to www.physiobalance.co.uk.

For any information on yoga classes or seasonal yoga teacher training please go to JulieHanson.com.

I wish you all the best and sincerely - have a great quality of life.

About the Author

A Fellow of the Royal Pharmaceutical Society, Elizabeth is an NHS and Health Council Award winning pharmacist. She is an Amazon Best Selling Author of 'Call the Pharmacist' and has a fortnightly 'Ask the Pharmacist' radio slot on RNIB's Connect Radio.

She can be heard from time to time on BBC Radio Scotland's Mornings programme commenting on health matters. Her Covid Diary 'The Other Frontline' is available on Amazon and her documentary of the same name can be found at www.nhsfrontline.com. Visit her website on erqualitylifesystem.com

You can buy her other books on Amazon and follow her on Facebook by going to www.facebook.com/CallThePharmacistUK.

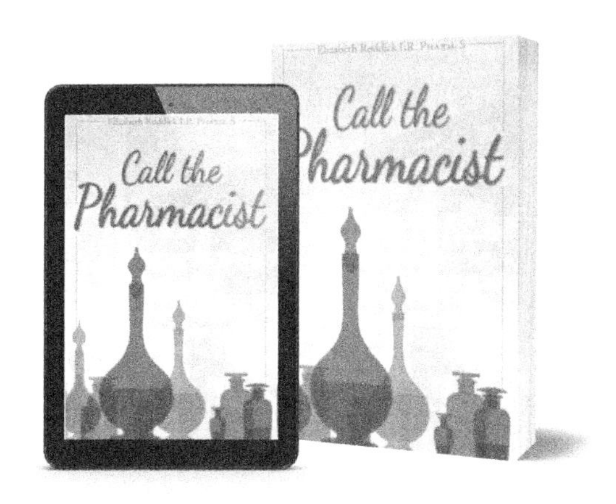

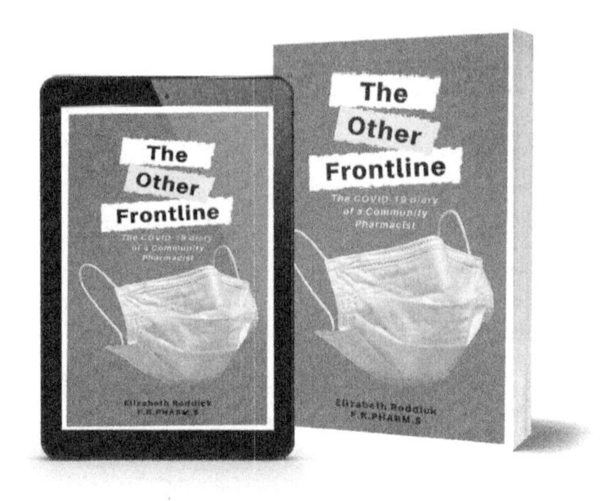

References

1 Andrade J.M. Drumond Andrade, F.C. de Oliveira, Y.A. et al. *Association between frailty and family functionality on health-related quality of life in older adults* Qual Life Res (2020).

2 Y. Henchoz, Fabiana Botrugno, +3 authors B. Santos-Eggimann (Published 2016) *Psychology, Medicine* Quality of Life Research 26, 283-289.

3 Bates method 'Better Eyesight without Glasses.'
4 Must A et al. *'The disease burden associated with overweight and obesity'* JAMA 1999;282;1523.

5 Funahashi Pschologia, 2011,54, 222-233.

6 Manninen et al Journal of Neuroscience 21 June 2017, 37 (25) 6125-6131.

7 Scientific Reports, 2015;5:16891 DOI: 10,1038/ step 16891.

8 David Feinstein '*The Psychology/Mental Health Category (for Personal Mythology)*'.

Printed in Great Britain
by Amazon